Confessions of a Trauma Nurse

Arayah Sunshine

CONTENTS

- **PREFACE** 5
- **DISCLAIMER** 6
- **THE GOOD** 7
- **NO HOPE** 8
  - NO HARM BUT FOUL ODOR 9
  - FREE 10
  - THE CHRISTMAS TEXT MASSACRE 11
  - SENSE 12
  - THE GENTLEMAN'S CLUB 13
  - SELF REFLECTION 15
- **THE BAD** 17
- **BURNS LIKE HERPES, STINGS LIKE A BEE** 18
  - HUNGRY AND AFRAID 19
  - NIC-KID 22
  - TUBE FEED MISHAP 24
  - LOWER 26
  - ROOM FOR AIR 28
  - THE UNSEXY NURSE 29
  - "FRED" 30
  - TOES: WHO NEEDS THEM? 32
  - MRI UPSET 33
  - THOUGHTS 34
  - NOW YOU SEE ME, NOW YOU DON'T 36
  - "THIS IS GOD" 37
  - I'M A LOVER NOT A FIGHTER 38
  - LUCKY SHOT 39
  - PASSION GAP WITH THE TWO-TONGUED WONDER 40
  - FRIENDS 41
  - GLORY SCRUBS 43
  - INSERT YOUR NAME HERE 44

LIFE ISN'T CHEAP	45
RAISE	46
FIRST IMPRESSIONS	48
NUMBERS	49
THE INTERNAL CUTTER	53
PINWHEEL	54
REPORT IS MORE IMPORTANT THAN YOU THINK	56
PUT A SOCK ON IT	57
CAN'T WIN	58
DEATH BECOMES HER	59
YOU'RE IN TROUBLE	61
WALK OF SHAME	62
ROOM C306	63
AN EYE FOR AN EYE	65
BLADDER BURST	66
BATTER UP	67
RODEO OF HORROR	68
SURPRISE	69
BED EXTENDER	71
MY APOLOGIES IF I OFFEND YOU	74
HOLES: EVERYBODY'S GOT ONE, RIGHT?	75
ANGEL	77
CODES	78
YOU GOT TO TAKE THE GOOD WITH THE BAD	79
BROKEN BONES AND SPIRITS	80
THE BLUE WAFFLE	81
THINGS NOT TO DO	82
CAUGHT WHITE-HANDED	83
SELFISH	85
THE FOREVER FORGOTTEN	87
EVERYBODY'S GOT A DREAM	87
DESPERATION	87
DISCHARGED FOR ETERNITY	88

GOT SALAD? 89
STIFF 90
DRIVING WHILE INEBRIATED 91
YEASTY BEASTY 94
BEST PATIENT QUOTES OF ALL TIMES 95
VANITY 96
NAKED AND AFRAID 97
DON'T BITE THE HAND 98
GREEN 100
EVERYBODY DOES IT 102
NO WORDS 104
WASTED EFFORTS 105
CHOOSE YOUR BATTLES WISELY 106
THE CRAIGSLIST GEM 107
TWO BIRDS, ONE STONE 109

THE UGLY 110
NEVER AGAIN 111
THE ONE-HANDED HIGH-FIVE 112
GOD VS. VANITY – NINE LIVES 113
THE UNANSWERED CALL OF DOOM 116
KINDNESS GOES A LONG WAY 117
GLORY 118
UNJUST 120
ONE IS THE LONELIEST NUMBER 122
SHAMMING DIDN'T NEVER HURT NOBODY 124
HAPPY FATHER'S DAY 125
PART I OF II: BALLS FOR DAYS 126
PART II OF II: BALLS FOR DAYS 128
CALL FOR YOUR STORY 131

PREFACE

The stories you are about to encounter are purely centered on truth. No names are used and parts have been changed to maintain confidentiality. All the stories are written in first-person but were derived from many trauma nurses and from many areas to preserve their privacy. As a nurse, you give a piece of yourself to every patient. For those of you in this field, this is something for you. A way of giving yourself a mental break from the broken, death, dying and the in-between. And yes, there is a difference between death and dying! Watching someone ooze out from multiple God-given and man-made orifices for months before they pass away is way different from breaking the ribs of a mother of three by doing chest compressions. You cannot save everyone from an inevitable death, but each one takes a toll on you. So yeah, my sense of humor is disturbed, crude and morbid and if that concerns you then you should stop reading now because you have been warned. The magnitude of the weight of our patients' worlds we bear on our backs is extensive and at times maddening. We engulf ourselves into each and every one of our patients' lives. We meet their family and friends, are with them for their most private moments and we hear the most touching aspects of their lives. We take all the bad from them so they can heal and recover. These are our stories.

DISCLAIMER

As much as you think one of these stories contains you or your brother's sister's cousin twice removed, I assure you it is not. I handle confidentiality with prime importance so all the stories have been changed to protect the privacy of all parties involved. Regardless that these events were all based on truth, the original stories will remain locked in my mind where they rightfully belong.

THE GOOD

NO HOPE

A young softball player had a terrible motorcycle accident. The doctors told her parents there was no hope and called in a company to speak with them about donating her organs. They immediately refused and insisted that she go to surgery. After having surgery to relieve the swelling on her brain she remained sedated for multiple days. Once she was extubated and the anesthesia wore off, she remained lifeless. A few days later, movement occurred. At this point, her body never rested and neither did her parents. We had to give her medication to at least slow her down, but sleep never happened. Her body moved constantly, her brain was in overdrive. But still, no communication, no fluid movements and the doctors continued to say there was "no hope." Her parents took turns watching over her, never leaving her side except for bathroom breaks. I would sit with her occasionally to allow them to sleep to make sure she didn't fall out of the bed or hit her head on anything. Parts of her skull were removed which left her brain vulnerable to the outside elements. Weeks went by and yet her eyes still wouldn't even track (aka follow a moving object). Nothing changed. Her parents continued to come and the bills piled up as they could not work because of their persistent involvement with her care. One day her mom was so tired she couldn't keep her head up, let alone her eyelids. It was like her neck was trying to cave in so I relieved her for a break to allow her to sleep. I needed to change the patient and get her washed up anyway. I was trying to be quiet to allow her mom to rest when she was suddenly startled by a loud familiar voice yelling "quit" and a subsequent swat at my hand. That's right, it's like her brain suddenly woke up and with an attitude at that. Shortly after, she was headed to rehab to relearn how to walk, among other things such as wiping and feeding herself. She excelled in her recovery and is now going to college on a full-ride scholarship for softball. No 'hope' never looked so good.

NO HARM BUT FOUL ODOR

A lady came in with a smell coming from her old foot wound that she had been caring for at home on her own. The doctor hadn't seen it yet. It smelled foul so I decided to change out the dressing since I wasn't immune to the smell yet. I gathered the supplies and was setting up shop when I noticed a noise. I couldn't tell where it was coming from so I shrugged it off. I placed a gloved hand on her foot to brace it to take off the dressing. Her foot vibrated. It felt like the thrill of an AV fistula (short for arteriovenous fistula which is a connection generally made surgically from an artery to a vein to aid in dialysis that makes a unique vibration). I peeled off the dressing to find a big pocketful of maggots. I asked her the normal questions one would ask if they found someone's old surgical site filled with critters and she informed me she didn't have feeling in her foot but she noticed an increase of flies in her house; so many she had to get a Venus fly trap. To be fair, I give her credit because they potentially saved her foot and life due to the gnarly infection she had going on that would have done tremendous damage that the maggots cleaned out.

FREE

A woman had been admitted to the hospital under police custody. In these instants, there has to be some form of observation. For those who are not conversant with such cases: depending on the county, after being arrested there has to be at least one police officer with the detainee at all times and that same county must pay for ALL the medical bills incurred while time is being served. This female was found face down alone in the jail in a room without cameras. There was no evidence of what happened. At this point, she could not move anything from the neck down. She had no history of seizures or back problems prior to this event. There were no wounds, dangerous objects and no evidence that would indicate foul play. Many tests were done, plus MRI after MRI to see if anything had been missed. Every test came back normal. I thought she was just trying to get a break from jail so I would occasionally come into her room as she slept and would poke her arms and legs but they never moved. The county was already paying for two police officers continuously to watch her, on top of the huge medical bills that were racking up. Weeks had gone by with no diagnosis, cause or cure. We couldn't send her out until we found something because the county was liable for her when this event happened and they didn't want to be at fault with a large lawsuit on their hands, beyond the medical bills that would continue to accumulate after years go by caring for a quadriplegic. Suddenly, the county threw in the towel and dropped all charges. Miraculously, hours later after the officers left, her arms moved. The next day she could move her legs and feet. By the third day, she was walking and discharged from the hospital. Had she still been there on the fourth day I would've almost bet money she would have walked on water.

THE CHRISTMAS TEXT MASSACRE

A city bus driver's bad wreck injured numerous people, including him. Both his legs had been broken in the crash and he was troubled by not being able to have a bowel movement. It had been well over a week since he had gone. We tried numerous tricks to make it happen, but there was also a psychological portion of it because there was no way to obtain access to the toilet due to his medical issues and lifting equipment failure. It had to be a bedpan. We are told our whole lives not to poop the bed and there he was trying to break this lifelong habit. Finally, success! After all that work on both of our ends (mostly his), there were multiple large hard lumps in the bedpan. His daughter was so proud of her father and how hard he worked that she took a picture. Her phone was low on battery so she used his to text herself the picture. It was one of those old flip phones and she wasn't familiar with it. She proceeded with the text with the caption of "best Christmas coal ever" seeing as though it was around the holidays. But she made a mistake. She slipped up and sent an all text, which sent this text to every contact there was in his phone. There were over 300 numbers just from his church alone. Plus, many from his personal life and work. The embarrassment was only half of it. His cell phone provider charged 40 cents per text going out and 40 cents coming in! As you can imagine if someone receives a strangely interesting poop photo from an injured friend, they are going to reply to it. The bill was MASSIVE. The patient felt so much better he didn't even care but he let her know quickly that it was her Christmas present.

SENSE

A woman came in with a nasty gunshot wound to the face. She placed a gun up to her chin and when she fired, the shot knocked her head back and it split her face apart. You could see everything. Luckily, her father was in the next room and called for an ambulance that just so happened to be in the neighborhood. She had to have an emergent trach because she had no place for air to pass through in and out. She was then rushed to the hospital and straight to surgery. It was a lengthy recovery filled with lots of surgeries, rehab and doctors' appointments. That day changed her life forever. She had a very interesting view about it and said that the bullet knocked some sense into her. She now writes self-help books and goes around the globe going from place to place as a motivational speaker. She tries to mostly to go to high schools and talk about the very sensitive subject of suicide. She is now in the high triple digits of the lives she has knowingly saved and counting.

THE GENTLEMAN'S CLUB

A gentleman had been in the hospital for over a month with three gunshot wounds to the chest. It was his first night on the step-down unit and he was so sad. He explained that he hadn't seen his kids in seven weeks because he didn't want them to see him like that. The ICU (Intensive Care Unit) would not allow him to have any visitors in the first place because no one knew who shot him and they didn't want an attempt on his life while in there during the investigation. He still had three chest tubes (a tube that drains fluid or pulls off air to allow for breathing to occur) in place; one on one side and two on the other with no end in sight at taking them out. He requested to have his best friend come by and insisted that his friend was not the one that shot him. After several pleas, I said he could stop by for an hour. Why not? It was Saturday night. What could go wrong? His friend came by shortly after and was happy to see him. I was doing my assessment and upon finishing I did as I always do and asked, "What can I do for you to make you more comfortable?" I guess he was feeling bold and squirrely with his friend by his side and exclaimed, "Strippers, we need some strippers." I told him, "OK, done." "No, no, no.... No ladies with any stab wounds or anything," he announced with a bit of worry as if he had dug himself into a hole he could not get out of. "You're one to talk, just trust me," I assured him. I did everything that I could to abide by his wishes like I do for all of my patients. I believe you should treat them no differently than your father, brother, sister or mother. You give them what they need, no matter the price because you do that for family and if you don't look out for them, who will? I had a friend that worked there who did not mind to go above and beyond to benefit the patient. I knew she would do it with very little convincing. She was a good dancer with a great sense of humor. Her price was 2 bucks and the ability to go home early. She went straight to his room, only grabbing a gown, cap, gloves and a mask to have items that she could reasonably take off. She barged in and busted a beat with her mouth to her dance removing her isolation getup piece by piece twirling them like a helicopter and tossing them in their faces. Money was flying everywhere. She saved her top end for last. Off came the mask and then the bonnet. They were chuckling before, but I thought I would have to fill out extra paperwork with them falling out on the floor laughing at the end. Oh, I forgot to mention this good caregiver made a pact with a separate patient that rendered her bald. The next day he made a miraculous recovery and was able to have all three chest tubes removed and was discharged within 3 days; worth every penny.

SELF REFLECTION

A young lady came in after being badly assaulted. She had been in the hospital for weeks in a coma after being beaten in the head to where brain matter could be visualized. She was so far gone that she would be placed in a nursing home since her body was considered stable, but no one was home. I came in to do frequent mouth care on her, but it was becoming increasingly difficult as she was moving a little bit. Her brain seemed like it was stirring. I tried to make time to bathe her using her own home soap and shampoo to help bring her back if she was still in there. Fun fact: Familiar aromas stimulate thoughts and memories. I grabbed my assistant to help me clean her up. Just after finishing her bed bath, I brushed her teeth. It needed to be done about every two hours because she had a trach and it helps to prevent any further issues. Suddenly, she woke up from her coma long enough to call me a bitch and go right back in it. Now, I'm OK with patients calling me that, but please don't leave any witnesses! My assistant helping me saw the whole thing. I was so embarrassed. Someone sprouting up out of a coma just to tell you about yourself must be telling the truth. It makes you question a few things. But she wasn't wrong for it. Just before she woke, I was trying to brush her beautiful rack of teeth. She was turning away and then she bit down on the toothbrush while raising her eyebrows up and down at me. At this point she was messing with me, so I knew she was in there. I told her she needed to let me brush her teeth because her breath must stink something awful. This was my fault as I suffer from word vomit occasionally. She didn't move another muscle for anyone else that day. The doctors said that it could have been a fluke and that she may never come back and if she did she would not function normally. The next night I bathed her with a different assistant in the early morning hours. We were singing to some music we heard on the tv that she must have liked because we looked down and there she was singing right along with us mouthing every word. We couldn't tell at first because her trach did not allow for much sound to come out unless she was furious and yelling. I told her where she was and what happened to her. She took it well. I asked her if she remembered calling me a bitch and she says as if in shock, "What... me... nooo." I couldn't help but laugh as she brought tears to my eyes because she was really there. No deficits. No long-term memory loss. She was all there. It took less than a week for her to be sent to rehab. The doctors were wrong. She made a full recovery. And as for me, I'm still a bitch. I'm just more aware of it now.

THE BAD

BURNS LIKE HERPES, STINGS LIKE A BEE

An elderly man was confused and needed to be changed. He had some dementia that was pretty far gone that left him unable to move much and he did not speak. I grabbed an extra pair of hands to help me check to see if he was clean and to turn him to prevent discomfort and pressure sores. As I was cleaning his man parts there were some red dots and a big spot of what appeared to be dirt. I was trying to be gentle in case it was sore. The dirt would not come off, so I rubbed it harder and faster. It still wouldn't come off, so I kept working. I'm in it to win it; I mean I'm sticking in there like a hair in a biscuit. Suddenly there was a rise and it's like the patient came to life saying, "Gentle as a butterfly, stings like a bee." Sure enough, I look down and there in my hand on his body part was a tattoo in the shape of a bee. It was just hard to distinguish when the skin was loose, plus the tattoo was undefined due to the apparent old age of the tattoo. The person helping me fell over the bedrail and into the bed laughing. I was not amused. It was about an inch short of a rub and tug.

HUNGRY AND AFRAID

A guy came in with multiple gunshot wounds. Having been shot by the police, he was on the news stating that he had only been shot once. Through the years, I've learned that you really can't believe what the news tells you in this business. As I was treating him, I got to know him. He spoke of how he fell on hard times and had been hungry. He went days without eating so his family could eat longer. He didn't have a penny to his name and stole some food from a grocery store even though it was against everything he stood for. He found steak reduced for a quick sale about to go bad since it would have been discarded if no one bought it. He figured it would not be missed and his family could have a meal they could enjoy. He was not experienced in the art of thievery as he had never stolen anything a day in his life. He had no clue on how to walk out with the goods without being noticed. He placed the meat up under his shirt and attempted to walk out when a bagboy observed him with a strange bulge. He ran and the employee chased him as if his job depended on it. Outside of the store stood an off-duty police officer in street clothes. The bagboy hollered for help as if he was wounded due to the exercise his body rarely saw. The officer took over the chase from there not knowing what he was even chasing him for and all the patient knew was that a different man from the parking lot was now running after him. The officer did not identify himself during the commotion. Suddenly the patient was backed into a wall with nowhere to go. The officer yelled at him to stop and bang bang. He was shot twice from behind for the love of his family. The news seems to leave those parts out. Here he was pouring out his heart and soul to me. He was kind, gentle, raw, social and loving. "I mean sure it was a ribeye but a man's got to eat." There wasn't a single angry bone in his body. He wasn't even upset with getting shot, he was only disappointed that he wasn't able to get the food to his family they so desperately needed and wouldn't be able to for some time.

Shortly after being discharged, he was met by the officer that shot him in the hallway. He arrested him right then and there. It was bad enough that he endured so much pain and was missing two fingers from the ordeal, but he was still being charged. I didn't follow what happened to him afterward. I assumed that he would have pled not guilty and would have a trial. When in fact he pled guilty and went to serve his time. More than a year later I was getting a report on a patient that had been there for a few days and refused to eat, drink and even talk. He was in police custody and handcuffed to the bed. I came into the room and removed his blanket hiding his face to find it was my old patient from the year before. He didn't look or act like his former self and appeared like he withered away. He saw it was me and spoke the first words he had spoken in over six months. Jail was not for him. He was a family man. He could not see his family and spoke of how he had been mistreated while incarcerated. He didn't want to share his burden but felt he couldn't take it anymore and planned to jump out a four-story window. That is how he came to be back in the hospital, broken again. The officers wouldn't even let him call anyone because they said that was a privilege he didn't deserve. So, I looked up his emergency contact information and called it while I was in his room to let him talk to his wife who didn't even know he was there. What was the officer going to do, arrest me? He got to talk to her for about twenty minutes while I was in the room. When he finished, I asked him why he wasn't eating. I remember it was one of his most favorite things to do if he had access to it. He explained that he never had an appetite anymore and his body was so used to going without for so long that it wasn't a big deal. Over the last year, he was only eating for survival. I asked him if there was anything that he was craving. He had to think long and hard about it. He came up with a particular soda and candy bar. The officer was not happy about this and I clarified that we were in my territory and it was happening. I promised him I would make it happen. I got my hands on the candy bar and give it to him, but the hospital did not carry the soda he wanted. I promised I would go to the store and bring him what he wanted when I came back on the next shift. The next day he was prematurely discharged shortly before I came back with the goods. Apparently, the officer made some excuse to the hospital doctor and said that he would be cared for in the jail in the infirmary. I worry that he may have had to pay for my stubbornness but at least he got to know a little kindness before going back.

NIC-KID

An elderly gentleman came in with a brain injury and significant underlying dementia. He looked just like Albert Einstein, hair and all. He was a mechanic the majority of his life and worked on a farm. He walked for numerous miles every day for decades and that didn't stop just because he was in the hospital with an injury. We could not keep him in the bed unless he was restrained and even then, that couldn't stop him. He was stable enough for rehabilitation placement, but he had to be out of restraints for two days, plus he was pretty sturdy on his feet so we set him free to move as he pleased throughout his room. We tried to allow him to have a personal assistant (sitter) to monitor him, but we were not capable of doing so under our staffing shortage. It was hard to redirect him because he was deaf and mute. It was like he was in his own little world and had been that way for some time. We brought in a guitar and he would come to the nurses' station and he would play it, take it apart and put it back together. That's right, a deaf man that played the guitar and sounded every bit of it. He had various items to keep his mind and body engaged. The man never slept, he was always tinkering with something. It's true, I worked four consecutive night shifts and he never slowed down. The day shift nurses said the same thing. It was impressive, and it takes a lot to impress a nurse. A few doors down there was a sweet beautiful girl I went to school with that came in for a broken arm. She was as shy and timid as a mouse with a heart of gold and manners for days. She was lying in bed while the doctor came in to speak with her and her mom. I mean really, out of 24 hours in a day the doctor is in there for about two minutes. During this two-minute block of time, this Albert Einstein lookalike came barreling through like a bull in a china shop and into her personal bathroom. He was something we call nic-kid with his socks on (translated to a person that is completely naked with the only exception for their socks). He then took the biggest, wettest dump this girl has ever heard, seen or smelled. What do you even do with that? He could have at least closed the door. The doctor, the girl and her mom were all mortified in disbelief.

TUBE FEED MISHAP

A very sick patient had a J/G tube (a double-lumened tube that is essentially a two-part system where one part goes into the jejunum and the other in the stomach that extends outside of the body to allow fluids to go in or out) that was clogged. I tried every trick in the book…. using warm ginger ale, a medication called Pancrelipase, a 10-mL syringe and my last resort which was Coke. As I was putting on as much pressure as I could, the other side of the tube gave way and shot gastric goo with a hint of Cola into the air. A fellow nurse popped into the room at the same time with her mouth hung open. It was a shot out of this world, straight into her mouth! The nurse still won't talk to me even to this day and someone told me she will never have Coke again. I bet you she will think twice before barging into a room again without knocking.

Am I the only one who likes to describe their patients' bowel movements using food to compare it to? Such as:

The long and narrow turd = a Snickers bar

The rabbit pellet= a Raisinet

The golf ball= a Malt Ball

The liquid= a chocolate shake to chocolate milk (depending on the consistency)

The paste=tooth paste

The solid unhuman baby= a whole can of busted cinnamon rolls

LOWER

I needed help turning a patient all the way up on his side because he wanted lotion rubbed on his back. He told me that with me being a female, I wouldn't have enough muscles to do the job so I needed to get a male with brute farm boy strength. I did as I was asked and grabbed the most muscular manly man I could find to help me. He got into a good position to hold the patient so I could baste this guy up with lotion. The patient then points at me and says, "not you" and shifted his lanky finger pointing towards my attractive co-worker stating "you." Ok, I thought, I'm off the hook. He helped me to push him over front facing towards me so I could hold him in place as he lubed up his backside. He started towards his neck when the patient moaned and he stopped. He explained that his skin was really dry and he couldn't reach it himself. The nurse told him, "That's fine but you don't have to make those noises." He said that he couldn't help it, but he would try to tone it down. The nurse obliged him and proceeded. He applied the lotion with the palm of his hand not wanting to touch him any more than he had to as the patient said, "Lower." The nurse went down about an inch. "Lower," he said as he went down another inch as the nurse was making a grossed-out face like he put something rotten in his mouth. This went on and on to where I was shaking holding his body in place. Both had their eyes closed, reminding me of the famous Sock and Buskin drama faces. The patient was overcome with joy and the nurse was overwhelmed with sweat, shame and a little bit of fear. Again, "Lower," he exclaimed, and the nurse yelped, "Man, any lower and I'll be checking your oil." In his defense, he was past the point of no return where he was exiting his back and entering new terrain, but his eyes were closed so he couldn't exactly tell. The patient's smile grew bigger and went for one more run, "Lower." The nurse opened his eyes and saw exactly where his hand was, threw his hands up in the air, exclaimed, "Oh, Hell, no," and marched out. The patient didn't care. He didn't even open his eyes or break his trance. I placed some pillows under him and walked out trying to maintain my composure. I busted out laughing as soon as I left the room and I was immediately greeted with a death stare. I told him, "Don't look at me, I didn't do it. There's nothing but grace, innocence, and beauty here." All jokes aside, I've never felt so much like chopped liver in my life.

ROOM FOR AIR

You ever get in real close to visualize for placement of a suppository just to be greeted with a huge gust of wind that blows your hair back? There are people out there that should have charged me for a perm for blowing my hair straight.

THE UNSEXY NURSE

I had a patient that was not thrilled about having a female nurse as he was gay and wanted me to "send in a sexy nurse." Being the nurse I am, I gladly obliged. I could not switch at that time, so for the next shift I hand-picked the next nurse that was geared more towards his liking. I might not have given a heads up when I said he wanted a bed-bath. When I came back in, I got a huge ear-full. I giggled about it for a bit and went on to business. At the end of that shift arose another opportunity. He needed to have lab work done. A female phlebotomist was about to go in. I stopped her dead in her tracks because there was a good-looking male phlebotomist with a thick New Orleans accent and a tan to go with it on the unit. I asked him to help me out and he graciously headed towards his room. That patient would think I was the 'Nurse of the Year.' I charted out in the hallway and almost forgot about the trap I had laid when he came rushing out. His face went past red and straight to purple. His eyes started to tear up, thinking he had done something wrong. His innocence was lost in that room. Apparently, he is one of those people that can't say no. He explained that the patient asked to grab the dark chest hair sticking out of his scrub top. He thought the patient was kidding so he said yes. The patient then grabbed hold of his thick patch of chest hair and pulled. He continued pulling to reel him in for a kiss. That's when he bolted. I feel a bit bad for setting him up and that instead of giving him the sympathy he needed, I asked him if his lips touched his or not. You can't be in the trauma profession and successfully make it without a sick sense of humor. Come to think about it he must have quit because I haven't seen him since.

"FRED"

So, leech therapy is a real thing that has been pretty successful at allowing people to keep their damaged extremities when we are pushing for a last-ditch effort to salvage it. Fun fact that I've noticed: most people who have leech therapy name each one of their leeches. Maybe in their minds it helps the patient to view them more as a pet than a parasite. Each one has to be killed afterward. Most folks view this as a sacrifice for the greater good. To do so, they must be soaked in alcohol. At this point, they purge all the blood they had taken in from the patient and die. One day I could find no alcohol so I assumed peroxide was the next best thing to do the trick. I grabbed a denture cup, filled it with peroxide, dropped "Fred" in, and watched him expel all the blood. I figured at this point I could just throw him away, so I chucked him in the trashcan. A few minutes later there was a huge bursting sound on the unit that sounded like an explosion. We walked around but couldn't figure out where it came from. It was so loud sound filled all the halls, but every room was in proper order. A few hours passed by and I was walking with the charge nurse. You ever have those moments when you walk past a room and you slowly inch back to look in because something was not right? Well, that was the case with the charge nurse and myself going past the leech room. The patient was asleep and the bathroom light was on. Upon closer examination, there was a thick red glossy line. Apparently, the loud bursting explosion came from the peroxide-filled denture cup I threw in the trashcan. Instead of dying, the leech climbed up the inside of the trashcan, down the outside of the trashcan, headed towards the bathroom where he must have lost the smell of blood and headed straight for the patient's bed to get back to finish his meal. He was climbing up the bedrail, approaching the sleeping patient when we found him. You could literally follow the trail because the journey was marked in blood.

"Fred" the leech was tough, resilient and hungry. The housekeeper was so pissed!

TOES: WHO NEEDS THEM?

You haven't really lived till you've pulled back a foot dressing only to discover an entire toe came off with it and without the patient even noticing. I've never known a single one to ever even feel it come off.

MRI UPSET

A guy came in with the worst smell my colleagues and I have ever smelled before and I have breathed in a lot of funk in my time. We played rock-paper-scissors to determine who would be the one taking care of him. I lost and headed to the room to do his admission history. He was irritated but who wouldn't be in his shoes? He had a knot on the side of his neck the size of a baseball. It was hard and clearly infected. He was ordered to have an MRI to determine how it could be approached because the mass had moved his anatomy around and if it got any bigger could block off his airway. Surgery was a success, but when he was greeted afterward it was not with a smile. The MRI revealed the top of an aggressive lung cancer. They let him know what was going on and ordered an MRI of his chest to see how far gone the cancer was so a treatment plan could be developed. The oncologist (the cancer doctor) spoke to him that night and let him know there was nothing that could be done for his cancer and he only had about a month to live. The next morning came and I thought he would be sad over the cancer news and maybe somewhat physically relieved by the pain. But no, he was furious. He was so angry he was shaking. He had just gotten off the phone with his insurance company. They would only pay for one MRI per year. He cussed out all the staff, called us every name you could think of and demanded that his second MRI be paid for. Sadly, he did not live to see his hospital bill.

THOUGHTS

Is it just me or do all the most stubborn patients do the best with head injuries because they are trying to prove the doctor wrong?

Memories:

You ever notice how sometimes no matter what happens, you can wash and wash, but the memory still remains?

Do yourself a favor and never give in to someone telling you that you need to smell something in the medical field.

It never ceases to amaze me the number of people that run themselves over with their own car or the number of people that think that it's ok to bring portable meth labs to the hospital.

Now I could understand being hit by a train once but being hit by a train three times is overkill. At some point, you've got to stop blaming the train and point your finger somewhere else.

Is it me or does every hospital unit have a person that breaks out in a musical seizure?

It seems that the fewer teeth you have, the more likely you are to wind up in the Emergency Room.

Is it bad to say that the more you piss me off the larger your catheters and your needles get?

Why are we grown adults in the medical field but some of us still think it's appropriate to flick boogers on the bathroom wall?

Don't you love when you are giving a patient a bed bath and they keep making sex noises even after their family busts in the room?

Why does it seem like nightshift and dayshift always have a beef with one another no matter where you go?

Don't you hate it when you walk through the hospital halls and make the mistake of having your mouth slap open? It's like you can practically taste the c. diff (something a person can get that causes massive diarrhea that smells horrific and is highly contagious).

Why are alcoholics so much fun?

The worst part about getting a female mule as a patient versus a male mule trying to smuggle or hide drugs that have burst and entered their system is that the woman can pack in twice as much like a loaded double barrel shotgun.

When the confusion clears up on patients that call 911 on the staff and accuse us of kidnapping and torture, I always like to ask them if they had to dial 9-911 to get out or did just calling 911 work? I like to remind them they owe me for that so now they should be on their best behavior.

NOW YOU SEE ME, NOW YOU DON'T

A man was admitted to the hospital for a self-inflicted gunshot wound to the face. It was his sixth attempt on his life but this one did a number on his quality of living. The impact of the bullet to his head caused so much pressure it caused his eyes to pop out from their sockets and dangle by the optic nerves. He would never see again. As for nursing care, he needed to have his wraparound gauze dressing changed multiple times a day to maintain moisture. It was as close to a once in a lifetime chance to see this kind of thing done as you would get. Naturally, I invited all the other nurses to this 4 am dressing change knowing he could not see them. I asked that they be wallflowers like a blossoming new student. I guess the Charge Nurse did not like this idea because she waited till they were all lined up in the room and paged everyone at the exact same time with the caption "That's what you get for trying to fool a blind man."

"THIS IS GOD"

There was a procedure that meant life or death for a patient. She was having some on and off hospital-acquired delirium and was extremely religious. She refused to have anything done until God spoke to her. In her right mind, she may have just done the procedure in the first place but she wasn't, so I gave her a little boost. I made sure she was awake and waited till she prayed. Timing is everything, you know, so I went on the call bell speaker and stated, "This is God." I told her she needed to get her procedure done or she would die and that it wasn't her time. I let a few minutes pass before I just so strolled by her room when she called my name to come in there. She had seen a bright light and God was there talking to her. She was just enough out of it to believe it was actually God speaking to her on top of there being not a single light on in her room. At least that's what I thought. Funny thing was, the joke was on me. It turns out that after I stopped speaking on the speaker the conversation continued. She told me that God spoke to her about doing the procedure but also about how there would be a small complication of bleeding involved but that she would be fine. She was completely awake, alert and oriented x4. I didn't think much of it, but she signed to do the procedure and that's all I needed. The next day she had her operation and she did great, but there was one small hurdle, a vein was accidently nicked and immediately repaired. It would cause her to go a little slower and rehab a little while longer but other than that she would be fine. Not too sure how ethical or moral it was but it saved her life in the end. So if it weren't for "God" stepping in she would not be alive today. The only thing that bothers me, though, is that everything that she was told by "God" after I stopped talking came true.

I'M A LOVER NOT A FIGHTER

Years ago, when our country was going to war a soldier received paperwork to send him to battle. He had joined in a time of peace and never thought he would have to go to battle. Plus, he was supposed to be a cook, not a warrior. He had to develop a plan. Unlike normal people that would have fled the country until the war was over and amnesty granted, this guy went one step further. He concluded that if he got rid of his trigger finger he could not defend with a rifle, rendering himself useless. Once the decision was made that he would sacrifice his finger for the greater good, he developed an idea. He arrived via ambulance bloody and missing a finger as planned. Everything was going well and according to plan. After he was cleaned up and stitched up he told me his story. I asked him his method of his finger disassembly and he said the quickest easiest way was to shoot it off. That's right ladies and gentlemen! He shot off the wrong finger. He still had to go to war but he just had to do so one finger shy.

LUCKY SHOT

A man was rushed to the hospital. A framing nail was lodged in his face and bleeding profusely. The CT scan of his head was incredible, one worth framing. It was lodged straight in his brain and sinuses missing everything vital that would have caused him major long-term problems. I knew there had to be a good story behind it, so I asked him about it after he got out of surgery and got back to his room. He explained how his nail gun misfired and stopped working. He then thought it was a good idea to look inside the exit point of the gun while having his finger still on the trigger. I got curious and leaned in close to ask a question burning inside of me. But before I could even say a word he exclaimed, "Hell yeah, it hurt." I heard that when you have a new serious head injury that it doesn't hurt and I really wanted to know. How did he already know the answer to my question before I even asked him? I am certain that nail made him a mind reader. No one will convince me otherwise.

PASSION GAP WITH THE TWO-TONGUED WONDER

A lady came in with an emergency. She was having trouble pleasing her husband because he told her she had gained too much weight. It was an emergency because she had to do something drastic to save her husband. She demanded to have her tongue split in two sections and for all of her upper and lower incisors (front teeth) to be removed to create a passion gap. We sent her home stating that it was not a true medical emergency. She then took matters into her own hands and created a real medical emergency. She went out to her car and took out her pocket knife. She drove the knife straight into the middle of her tongue and pulled until there were two pieces of her tongue instead of one. She knew that we had to help her now and she was right. We stopped the bleeding, numbed her up and stitched both pieces back together. She did all that for only some permanent numbness. Her husband was upset that he had to stop his date with his new girlfriend and come to sign paperwork that she refused to sign. He was so upset he left her right then and there. That was fine, I guess, but he didn't have to bring his girlfriend in the hospital room to do it. Rude!

FRIENDS

A lady was admitted to the hospital due to a small car wreck. There was nothing different that stood out about her. She was kind, timid and sweet. As the night went on she requested to have no visitors because she wanted to rest. That was no problem, so I arranged that for her. The next night I worked she said she changed her mind and asked if she could have her visitor restriction lifted to restricted visitors only. Again, no big deal as she never asks for anything and is always so quiet and polite; hence I didn't mind changing that for her. She wanted her boyfriend to come see her, so I put him on the list. He came by and left shortly after. The next day as I was getting a report on her, I asked if her boyfriend stopped by again, and the nurse said, "You mean girlfriend." "No, I mean boyfriend." Her boyfriend appeared to be pretty manly; I don't know how the other nurse mistook him for a girl. After finishing the report, I went in to say hi and there she was in the bed with another girl. She introduced me to her and her eyes were basically telling me not to say anything. I did my assessment and she told her girlfriend that the nurse needed to have privacy to do what I needed to and that she would have to go. I went along for the ride with her story. Once the girlfriend left, she explained that she had a girlfriend and a boyfriend that didn't know about each other. I mean, I had come to that conclusion without her having to tell me, but she said that her strategy to keep them separate was to have her come by in the daytime and him come at night as they have opposite schedules regardless. Just then her boyfriend knocked on the door and came in. I had trouble looking at him in the face, so I quickly exited out. As I was on my way down the hall I saw her girlfriend come through walking fast. She saw me as she blew past saying she forgot her phone. I guess I could have stopped her, but I didn't. She popped in the door without knocking. I stood in awe for a few moments as you can imagine there was much to be said. The talking rapidly turned into yelling.

As I called security, the yelling stopped for a moment and the boyfriend left. The yelling revived again and ended in a door slamming with the girlfriend stomping away in tears. That night, the patient stayed on her phone and was so upset. I didn't know what to do so I just kept on checking up on her. I checked on her one last time at about 5 in the morning and there were three people in the bed; the patient, her girlfriend and her boyfriend. He had the cheesiest grin on his face as he looked up at me and proudly stated, "What can I say, my girl's got a girlfriend."

GLORY SCRUBS

It's always good practice to bring in another person with you if you can when you are putting in a catheter. I had a man that was in a terrible accident that left him essentially a vegetable. He looked perfect on the outside, but nobody was home on the inside. There was nothing we could do for him besides feed him, turn him and clean him. He sometimes peed on his own and sometimes didn't. I just kept an eye on him and scanned his bladder to check for urine residual every few hours to keep him comfortable. He had been doing well with urination for the most part until I scanned him and he had a high triple-digit amount of urine in his bladder. It was late, and I still had a ton of stuff to do so I grabbed my assistant and scurried in. I gloved up, took a strong hold of his man-part and as soon as I encroached the tip of his anatomy a strong stream of liquid gold blasted out. I turned it away from me as fast as I could, and the CNA jumped back with wild eyes glaring at me. He pounced fast like a panther. I then threw away all of the supplies and went on my merry way to chart. A while later I was coming to an end on my charting and noticed something was off. My CNA was wearing the scrubs of glory (the uniform you can get from the hospital if yours are soiled from bodily fluids). I had an instant epiphany. "I peed at you!" I was so busy and focused on my work I didn't realize that when I was saving myself from an explosion of urine, I sacrificed my CNA. I peed all over him using someone else's pee stick. Anyway, that's the way my mind viewed it as I slipped up and announced, "I peed at you" in front of all my co-workers. Sadly, that saying didn't go away for months.

INSERT YOUR NAME HERE

One of my favorite things to do is if a patient likes to scream, I like to insist they scream out certain names of people that are working on that shift. It may not seem like a big deal to you but when someone hears their name being screamed out repeatedly for 12 hours straight, that person gets a tad unhinged by the end and it fills my heart with joy to watch them unravel as the shift goes on.

LIFE ISN'T CHEAP

As you may know, many homeless people have mental illnesses. Those that cannot function in this world must find other means of survival. Sometimes there are some that are desperate enough to put themselves in harm's way. It may be because they are hungry, hot, cold or even just tired of the elements. A man came in because he threw himself in front of a moving car on the coldest day of the year. The car did a slight grazing tap only on his body. There was no actual impact and no injury. We still had to run test after test. MRIs, CTs, x-rays, ultrasounds, lab work, etcetera. He professed that he was paralyzed from the waist down. He had no job, no insurance and no place to go. He was going to see this thing through. He had multiple friends come in and shower leaving years' worth of dirt and debris behind. The smell was atrocious, and he had so many people stay the night that there was hardly any room on the floor to walk. I would go into his room while he slept and jab at him to see if his feet moved. They did. He was faking and there was nothing that we could do about it. After weeks of being in the hospital, he became accustomed to us waiting on him, taking care of him and tending to his every need. Since he never got out of bed, he became very dependent on us. One day the hospital had to free up a bed because it was full and new trauma patients waited for care. We reached out far and wide, but no one would take him. We couldn't legally put him on the streets, so they paid for an apartment for him and a private investigator to go with it. He only knew about one of the two because the day he rolled up in a wheelchair was his first and last because he stepped right out of it and made a miraculous recovery that the hospital would not flip the bill for. This guy actually answered the door on his feet and about hit the floor when he was greeted with his quarter of a million-dollar hospital bill.

RAISE

A woman was in a terrible rock-climbing accident. She broke both of her legs in multiple places. Her legs weren't the main problem, though. Her major issue was her hemophilia (a blood disorder where the blood fails to clot in one of the sequences of events that must happen for blood to clot). There are nine different factors that could go wrong with clotting and each and every one of them have to be administered through an IV continuously until the person is not at risk for bleeding anymore. This lady had three of the nine factors that had to be corrected for her to properly heal and not to die from blood loss as she would have continued bleeding out. Now you would think if you knew that you had a problem that could kill you from a cut if you didn't get to a hospital fast enough, you would live a simple life. Not this lady, she was living on the edge. Her ailment made her feel most alive when she was doing something that had the potential of killing her. Her insurance had dropped her more than a decade before because of her hemophilia combined with her risky behavior. She was in poor health in the first place. I don't see how she could have climbed up even one set of stairs, let alone a mountainous cliff. She must have lost her mind. The kicker is this was her third time almost dying and being admitted for the same thing; falling during a rock climb. Because of this, the hospital had to flip the massive bill and had to cut out a few things like bonuses, raises, new employees and PTO (paid time off). She was nice, but not nice enough to be out of a raise. That meant that thousands of people did not get a merit raise or a cost of living raise for three years. We need our money. That's how we put food in our mouths and a roof over our heads. Money shouldn't be why we are in this profession but that's our livelihood. The entire hospital system was unable to see a raise. When all the prices were going up around us, our revenue of income remained the same no matter how good of a job we were doing. I had co-workers that were having their electricity turned off, applying for food stamps and getting foreclosure notices in the mail and placed on their front doors. This one person affected thousands of people in a negative way. There are many people in the US who live from paycheck to paycheck and it hurts to go without, especially when you work so hard to be where you are in this field. I almost felt bad for her when we had a heart to heart one day. She expressed that she felt like if she stopped breathing that no one would save her, which is not true. We would do whatever it takes to save a life, no matter whose life it is and as long as they want to be saved. The ugly part is that she couldn't wait to get some money up and get out the hospital to buy more equipment and get back to climbing again.

FIRST IMPRESSIONS

The ICU was full and one of the ICU beds was needed desperately which meant that the least sick person had to transfer to the step-down unit. The man they sent was bad off. Almost all of his ribs were broken, his spleen was removed, a colostomy bag placed, multiple drains placed for pockets of infection, plus he had a chest tube and a trach. With these injuries, it's like he had one foot in the grave and the other foot on a banana peel. He was transported over almost when I was told that he was coming. I could hear the stretcher approaching so I immediately went straight to his door to greet him. You only get one shot at a first impression you know. Just before entering his room I introduced myself and he stopped me with his hands. He was wide-eyed and appeared worried and restless. He was trying to speak but nothing came out. I'm thinking this guy will tell me something life altering like he can't breathe or has a sense of impending doom type of thing (where someone has a feeling that death is fast approaching and eminent). He keeps adamantly pointing down with such anxiety and concern. We hadn't even made it into to the room yet. He was literally outside of his new room in the hallway not letting us go. He couldn't speak due to his trach, but he kept mouthing something. By this point, all the staff on the floor is trying to help because generally if you see a mound of nurses somewhere there is a problem and we help each other in any way that we can. He continued pointing at me then pointing down towards his backside. Maybe something was poking him but I couldn't see it or feel it, so I had some people help me turn him over and lift his gown up and there it was. He may as well have just smacked me in the face. He got me and he got me good. There it was plain as day, a tattoo that read "your name" smack dab on his back end. Everyone on that side helping me saw it so I couldn't pretend I didn't see it. He pointed at me yet again mouthing what he had been but only this time it was clear "your name's on my ass".

NUMBERS

An elderly homeless man was admitted with several rib fractures and a brain bleed after being hit by a vehicle because he thought it was a good idea to sleep in the middle of the road. He was a paranoid schizophrenic and trusted no one with his name. By law, we cannot refuse care so we just called him Rumpelstiltskin. Rumpelstiltskin came to trust some of us to a certain extent. Though, he had some weird thing with numbers he could not trust. We couldn't even write the date in his room or have any phones where he could see them because they have numbers on them. Numbers just freaked him out. I figure everyone's got their one thing. His was numbers. He eventually got better physically, but could not walk and wouldn't be able to for some time. Because of his mental illness, unknown identity, lack of funds and insurance, he was rejected by all the surrounding rehabs and nursing homes. We all pitched in and got him a tent and some clothes. The hospital was generous enough to give him a wheelchair and a cab ride. Upon discharge, he was so thrilled that someone cared enough for him to replace his worldly possessions that were probably gone. Within two days of being discharged, he was found in a local public bathroom laying on the floor in a pool of urine, feces, and blood (hopefully his own). He was sent back to the hospital via ambulance confused, dehydrated and hungry. The EMS crew was kind enough to bring his belongings with him. As I inventoried his things I noticed that there was something on his tent. He thought so highly of us that he felt the need to label the stuff we bought for him with his name; his real and God-given name. It seemed wrong to call him something else after all this time, so he still let some of us call him by the name we had known him by for months. The social worker did digging and came to discover he had a brother. He gave us permission to speak to him, but he could not talk to him because it takes numbers to dial a phone. The brother had something very interesting to say. Rumpelstiltskin was in the military for some time and retired from there with full compensation. Once his mental illness worsened, his brother became his power of attorney and got him declared as disabled. He set up an account that had both avenues of income streaming in; about $5,000 a month. That was almost a decade ago. He had more money in his account than some people will ever see in a lifetime. He went to the best rehab money could buy, but he told us before he left that he preferred his tent.

Nurses Got Jokes:

A very long-term patient had an unhealthy infatuation with me as I was in his room a lot tending to his needs. When I could escape from there, we nurses used to have this thing we did every Monday where we would go through the Missed Connections section on Craigslist amongst other things during a short amount of downtime to decompress. One week in going down the list there was a submission that read something like this: "As you gracefully yet forcefully placed the catheter into me, I gazed into your starry eyes and for the slightest moment in time my heart stopped and all I could see was you and I. The image became clearer. It was like the scene from the movie 'Dumb and Dumber' where you were driving a moped and I was in the side car riding alongside you with a trail of snot going down my face from each side of my nostrils. I knew then that we were a match made in Heaven. Forever yours, Patient 0". My ruthless co-workers attempted to make me think it was the patient of mine that I called my hospital-acquired boyfriend. Each and every one of us has one. You know the one, the patient that is a thorn in your side because they are like an infection you just can't get rid of.

The nursing staff and I had a thing going that we deemed as quarter after laughter. You know that moment when you are working nightshift where both your brain and your body decide that you should be asleep, and everything is quiet but you can't. We try to keep people awake by using humor and scare tactics. I know, I know, we are basically educated toddlers with cash, but it works for us. It's not exactly politically correct but it saves us from being sleepy on the job which can lead to an unsafe environment.

We do things like:

Hide in a corner and wait in a high traffic area to squirt someone in the downstairs privates and we call them swamp crotch for the rest of the night

Place a bucket of water on top of a cracked door that is not a patient's room.

THE INTERNAL CUTTER

A man came in for the same thing he is always admitted for; swallowing knife blades. That's right, knife blades. Whenever he was stressed out or had some big mishap in his life, he would go to the kitchen, take the handles off the kitchen knives and swallow them. He is what I call an internal cutter. Each blade he swallowed made him feel better. He also had a thing where he would stick objects in his pee hole (or urethra for all those technical folks out there) so he always had to be monitored under close supervision while in the care of the hospital. He liked to stroll around the unit and people watch. One day directly in front of the nurses' station he fell to the ground and convulsed. I thought to myself, 'Shit, he's either gotten something stuck inside somewhere that doesn't belong or those knife blades have finally caught up with him'. It was shift change so there were tons of extra people there that rushed to his rescue and a code was called overhead to bring more help from outlying teams. He had been there long enough he didn't have any IV access, plus he was a very difficult stick from the decades of IV drug abuse (continued insertions of needles can change the dynamics of the veins and leaves them unviable for future IV use). We had to get access to give him meds and we had to get it fast. A few minutes without oxygen to the brain and proper medications is the difference between life and death. The IV team person was busy trying to work his magic on him with poor veins and a moving target when someone in the large crowd warned "be careful, he has AIDs. Unexpectedly the convulsing body on the floor exclaimed, "I don't have AIDs, I'm having a seizure." The attentive crowd immediately dispersed going in all directions from which they came. Anyone that has been in this business long enough knows that if you can talk, you are not having a seizure. A seizure renders you speechless. It was all an elaborate scheme to get something I call "AA": attention and Ativan.

PINWHEEL

A very sick gentleman was forced to be detained in the hospital because of a faulty valve in his heart due to long-term IV drug abuse. He was deemed incompetent and unable to make his own decisions because of his poor life choices. All he wanted to do was leave the hospital and go back to his street drugs. He tried everything he could to break loose from the clutches of the hospital, like sneaking out, getting a lawyer and saying what he thought we wanted to hear to get him out of there. None of which worked, he was stuck there until he was healthy enough to have his valve replacement surgery. He had a visitor come in and the sitter (a hospital companion that continuously monitors a patient for safety) didn't think much of it because all the visitors for this patient were mandated to be searched prior to coming into the room. I saw the person enter the room and decided to greet them for shits and giggles. As soon as I walked through the door, the visitor was handing the patient a box of baked goods. We live in a day and age where not too many people go out of their way to bust out the roller, open their oven and bake a made from scratch pastry. I looked in the box out of sheer curiosity and noticed some strange crystals. I grabbed the package from the patient and marched it straight down to the nursing station. It turns out that this visitor took the time to carefully construct a pinwheel masterpiece baked with love and meth. I feel like I shouldn't complain because he made a point to offer me some.

Items thrown at me:

Semen

Poop

Cheap phones-never the expensive kind

Call bell

Telemetry monitors as big as an old box TV

Tampons- sometimes new, sometimes used

Hot, wet burp all up in my face and that's not exactly a part of the classification but if you've ever worn it like a mask then you would think it should be too

A cast

REPORT IS MORE IMPORTANT THAN YOU THINK

There was a new policy just implemented at the hospital where I work to cut down the time a patient had to wait in the Emergency Room. The policy mandated that once a room was decided upon for a patient you have only five minutes to prepare everything before that patient arrives. I was elbow deep and fifteen minutes into a forty-five-minute dressing change when I got a five-minute warning page (and yes, some of us still use archaic beepers). I scurried to tape up what I could on that patient so I could finish later. By the time I got out of that room I didn't have much of a chance to go through the next person's chart because of the tight time constraints when "squeak, squeak, squeak." There they were. I rushed to greet the patient and nurse at the door since they didn't have to even call for a report when I laid eyes on the patient. Half of her face was up, and the other half hung down. There had to have been a two-inch difference. No kidding. This person was on the Trauma floor, but from the looks of it needed to be in the ICU receiving lifesaving measures due to a stroke. I tried to play it off all smooth like using my poker face and calmly asked, "What brings you here?" She looked at me with her one good eye as the other one dragged along trying to keep up and said, "I'm having a... what's it called... a heart attack." The nurse with her bent over and said, "You mean a stroke." "Yeah, that's it," she exclaimed. The nurse with her didn't even know what she was truly there for. He said he was just transporting her. Somebody needed to say something because that just wasn't good enough for me or that patient. This lady would not die on my watch and just as I hung my mouth open to politely go off on the nurse while trying to figure out what we were going to do, the patient points at me and says, "Ha, I'm just shittin' ya." Had I gotten a report they would have told me she was there from a fall but to watch out because she is a jokester.

PUT A SOCK ON IT

I couldn't help but get frustrated with my patient as I entered the room and he was receiving fellatio from his wife. That part of it didn't bother me so much. What got to me was the fact of him knowing what time I was coming into the room to do paperwork we previously agreed on together with his wife included and they are very timely people. Last, he had been there over a month and had not showered, groomed, bathed or even so much as ran a rag down there the entire time and he reeked every bit of it.

CAN'T WIN

A lady decided to commit suicide. To build her confidence up enough to do it, she decided to get drunk. She would not shoot herself and she had no pills that would do the job, so she chose to swallow antifreeze. Later she admitted herself to the hospital sick, vomiting blood and furious that she was still on this earth. Apparently, the only antidote for antifreeze is alcohol.

DEATH BECOMES HER

I was taking care of a slow code (a person that is a full code but should not be, such as someone who had a DNR living will but the family fights to keep them alive despite their wishes). She was well over 100, demented for decades, and had multiple severe pressure ulcers past the bone, fed through a tube, unable to move, contracted and in constant excruciating pain. Her family wanted her to stay alive at all costs so that they could continue to collect her disability and pension checks. She was on a monitor that sounded off when her heart rhythm went from somewhat normal to asystole (where the heart stops beating). I finished my sandwich, told the secretary to call the funeral home to pick her up and began to slowly walk to her room. Her jobless, inebriated caregiver great-granddaughter just so popped up at the exact time I arrived and made sure that I did everything my team and I could. After an hour and a half of chest compressions and breaking every rib, she had multiple occasions that she was able to keep a heartbeat going on her own for a short amount of time. We eventually saved her and it felt like shit. Her body was here and her mind was far gone just like the great-granddaughter who had to leave to fill her pain prescriptions even though great-grandma's drug screen was negative and she would probably not leave the hospital alive. It was gloomy in the room. Maybe it was the dim lights, all of our shame for actually helping her to make her heart beat longer or maybe it was the spirit leaving her body. Suddenly a dark presence entered the room. He wore all black: black hat, black hoodie and black pants with a black stretcher and body bag. "I'm here to get the body," he exclaimed. Was I actually seeing the Grim Reaper, or had I done too many chest pumps? It was the transporter for the funeral home. I asked him to step outside the room so I could gather my thoughts and try to stabilize and comfort her. Clearly, she was not dead and he knew it but waited anyway. I exited the room after about 45 minutes. He was still there. "Well, I haven't got all day," he stated as he pointed at her when abruptly the monitor went off again signaling her heart had ceased to beat. There she was dead. A chill went up my spine and I had goosebumps all over. The doctor was at the nursing station coming towards me shaking his head. We would not put her through that again. Shortly after pronouncing death, I assisted to move her fragile body over and observed something. When leaning over I noticed his name badge, "G.R.".

YOU'RE IN TROUBLE

Have you ever been forced to quickly move a patient from a bed to a stretcher? I was assisting a lady that needed to be transported via ambulance and the EMTs (Emergency Medical Technicians) had no time to spare. EMTs are always fast paced and have a sense of humor that is a different kind of funny. I was rushed to where they did not give me time to put my gloves on. They were stronger than me, so the two of them pulled on one side while I pushed. At the end of their count to three, they ended up pulling me along with the patient. Here I was sprawled across this woman's huge fresh, warm mound of pee and poop with my hands and arms covered. The EMTs started to laugh and sing "you're in trouble" but the way the song was sung sounded like "ur-in trouble." That's one thing you'll do just once and never again.

WALK OF SHAME

You know you've had a bad day when you've worn four types of body fluid and you carry a smell with you for each and every one. You may change your clothes but that doesn't always help and you may not be able to tell where it's coming from. There is no such thing as going home or taking a shower until your shift is over.

ROOM C306

I took care of a gentleman for three consecutive nights. He had extensive belly surgery and could not move around much as his incision could not be closed due to swelling. His intestines could pop out with minimal effort because there was nothing more than a dressing holding his internal contents in place. We had meaningful conversations and spent a fair amount of time together as I cared for him during my shifts. About midway through the third night, he tells me that his wallet fell. He started to climb onto the floor to look for it. I stopped him dead in his tracks as he was not going to have to go to surgery on my watch to put his newly outside bowels back inside of him. I bent over to look under the bed, but I saw nothing. He went on and on about how he needed his wallet right then and there. He said that if I didn't find it, he would just get it himself after I left the room. So I did it. I took the plunge. I got down on that contaminated hospital floor. I don't care how often they sanitize it, it'll never be clean in my eyes; at least, not enough to do what I was doing. I've seen too much. Now I don't get on my hands and knees for nobody, but he had me feeling like a hostage and crouched over like a wounded animal. As I was pressed up against the gritty floor, he goes on to say he had two hundred-dollar bills that turned into butterflies and fluttered away. Oh, hell no! I was beyond frustrated before but I was pissed at this point. He was messing with me. I had been with him for three nights and never even had a clue that he was about four types of crazy to put me on the floor like that. I turned his bed alarm on to a higher sensitivity and marched out. Once I regained my composure I went back in the room to figure out what was going on to make him say some off the wall stuff like that. After I got over myself and cooled off, I approached him, but he didn't want to tell me what was bothering him. I told him that I'd be back and we could figure it out from there. Later, I was standing outside of his door doing some charting before I came in and I could hear his voice. He was upset and telling someone to go away. I rushed in and found him alone and his phone across the room. "Who were you talking to?" I asked. "No one," he said. He sounded nervous and worried. After some nudging, he finally told me there was a man at the end of his bed wearing a strange hat and overalls. Clearly, there was no one there and he knew that, but he seemed real to him. The weeks passed by and his visions just got worse. He was yelling and jumping out of bed because of his mind but this did not do well with his body, which extended his stay. Something happened one day where the water stopped working in his room and he had to move. Almost as soon as he changed rooms he perked up. The hallucinations were gone, his body seemed rejuvenated and he was healing properly. Most of us chalked it up to timing for his new psych meds to work. Once the water was restored the room opened back up and a young female was placed in it. Her second night being there she spoke of a nightmare she had of an outdated dead train conductor sitting at the end of the bed. She tried to get out of there as fast as possible and discharged the next day. On and off for months patients in that particular room, C306 , saw a man at the end of the bed. All had similar descriptions. He never tried to harm anyone or speak, he was just there. The last person to see him claimed to be a psychic. She said she needed help to move a spirit on. We claimed that we didn't know what she was talking about, but she knew that we knew good and well exactly who she was talking about. She had a friend come in with a few items and they performed some type of ritual. No one ever spoke about the man in the overalls again but before the psychic left, she told a few fortunes. Most were generic but one of the staff members she said would be dead within the year. That was eight months ago and he is still holding strong.

AN EYE FOR AN EYE

I had worked with the same gentleman for four twelve-hour shifts in a row. He had an emergent belly surgery that required him to have an NG tube (a tube that extends from the nose to the stomach) that needed to be hooked up for continuous intermittent suction and occasionally unhooked for medications and ADLs. I spent hours in that room talking with the patient and getting to know him. He had one strange thing though; he always had a big jar of Vaseline on his bedside table. Over the years I've learned not to question certain things and that's one of the instances where I draw the line. It was 4 am and I needed to check the output of his NG when something didn't seem right. I felt like something was looking at me. I looked around. The patient was asleep and snoring away. I looked around more. There it was. On the table right by the Vaseline laid an eyeball. No way! There is no way I have taken care of someone for almost 48 hours in four days and not noticed a fake eye. So I got closer, and closer, and closer, but still couldn't tell. It was dark and I didn't want to wake him up due to my now questionable assessment skills, so I reeled in closer. I was within an inch of his face and sure enough, I was staring at a sunken place where an eye should be. Suddenly a rough, abrasive voice shouted, "Well either kiss me or get out my face." I'll be more inclined to look my patients in the eye more closely and use a light to check for irregularities from here on out, even with belly issues.

BLADDER BURST

I was charting I&Os (intake and output) for my shift and realized I had a patient that hadn't peed all night. It was eleven hours into my shift and 6 am. I had to hurry before shift-change so I could attempt to leave on time. The patient had trouble peeing in the past so I brought the bladder scanner in with me. He said he didn't have the urge to pee and that was not an option for me. That pee was going to come out one way or another whether he gave it or I had to get it. Being the thorough male nurse I am, I palpated (manually feel) for his bladder. It was impressive how big and rock hard it was. I never felt anything like it. Could it have been a tumor causing his urination troubles? I continued to press on him and asked him if it hurt with me touching there. I looked up and he had his hands interlocked behind his head with a huge cheese-eating grin on his face. That wasn't a bladder at all! I ran out the room furious. That man's bladder could burst before I stepped foot in that room again.

BATTER UP

I've gotten so good at what I do that when I give meds and the patient spits one out I'm usually able to catch it in midair in the nick of time. Typically, they are so shocked with the element of surprise they wind up taking the pill anyway.

RODEO OF HORROR

A man came in with a head injury that caused a significant amount of confusion with a false sense of reality. He was so frustrated about not being able to smoke that he was fidgety, having tons of tantrums and acting out. He acted out so much that we had to restrain him. His wrists and ankles were strapped up, but do you think that stopped him? No! Do you know what this man did with his time? He had nothing better to do than yank on his catheter until he pulled it out even with the restraints on. Mind you, a catheter empties urine directly from the bladder and out the body and is held in place by a fairly large balloon. Luckily, we have this thing we do where if someone is just off enough that they think a candy cigarette is real we give it to them. I grabbed a pack of the candy cigs from my locker, gave him one and lit it up using the Zippo app on my phone and even let him blow out the flame for good measure. When he was busy with that we cleaned up all the blood and urine off the floor, ceiling, and walls as it wasn't enough for him to self-remove this thing. Once it was out he felt the need to pretend he was in a rodeo and was trying to lasso a bull. As you can imagine there was bodily fluid everywhere. It looked like something straight out of a horror flick. He smoked one for everybody on the floor that night.

SURPRISE

We all look into the patient rooms as we walk by. It's the same sights over and over and over again. It is very rare to ever get surprised. One day I was coming back from buying dinner from the cafeteria when I walked past something that didn't seem right, so I slowly backed up and peeked in the door. The patient was in a veil bed (a breathable tent-like apparatus that goes on top of the hospital bed to avoid falls). Looking in further, I could see the patient. He was climbing the sides of the net as if he were a monkey surrounded by a cage at the zoo. And there it was; the smell. It was like being smacked in the face by a hot, sopping wet, dirty diaper. There was poop in the net. Poop in the bed. Poop on the rails. Poop on the floor. Poop caked everywhere! And then it happened. He saw me see him. That was a mistake. He stared at me right in the eyes. I should've looked away, but I didn't. Without blinking or breaking his stare at me he then took both hands grabbed a pile of his own excrement, double-fisted it and proceeded to finger paint his face with it like he was a warrior. That's one war I was willing to lose. Some things you just can't unsee. So, what do I do? I did what any good nurse would have done in my shoes. I gracefully shut the door and headed to my original destination. The damage was already done. There was no backtracking. It's not like ten minutes would make that much of a difference for him but it would for my food, so I went to finish what I started. His nurse was in the break room eating. I sat down with my hot food and ate, making small talk. It would be rude of me not to let her finish eating her food first before her world came crashing down and her innocence lost. I figured she'd get more bang for her buck if she threw up because then she would've tasted her food twice over. As she finished her last bite I let her know her patient in E612 wanted to see her. She came back almost as soon as she had left but this time she was flaming. Knowing that I had been eating for about ten minutes before saying anything, she yelled, "You knew about that and didn't say anything?" There was no getting out of the grave I had just dug for myself. She made me help her do the cleanup which really needed about six more people. He really popped my cherry on that one because I don't get too many firsts these days.

BED EXTENDER

I took care of a gentleman for three nights in a row. He was so tall that he was bent up and scrunched in the bed. His legs couldn't even straighten out and his head was completely on the wall. I tried to get him a bed extender to give him an extra foot and a half, but the entire hospital was out. "No worries," he would say. He just looked so uncomfortable, plus he had a nasty leg infection that had been brewing for a while. I got a call one night from the pharmacy to make sure his weight was correct because they were specially formulating his antibiotic to his size. The pharmacist asked, "Well how big is he because he looks to be a big boy by these numbers." I told him he was not out of the ordinary and was of normal build and stature. I went on into his room and found him sleeping. I was told by the doctor to apply pressure on his leg to allow some of the infection to ooze out and his pain to ease up as he was requiring way more than your average Joe for pain meds. He was heavily medicated with narcotics so the nursing staff could relieve the pressure from his infection. I dived in for the chance to put the squeeze on this thing like any other nurse would do in my situation with a good pimple ready to be popped dangling in front of his/her face. So I quietly put my gloves on and went to town. It was so awesome, like a volcano erupting! It was so awesome until it wasn't anymore because he was awake staring at me getting busy on his leg. "We talked about this, you knew it was coming," I said. "I know, but you don't have to enjoy it so much" he exclaimed. I tried to put my poker face back on and keep it moving but he said it was too painful to do anymore. I let him off the hook and told him that we'd try again later because that is the main thing that could give him some fast relief. The weekend came to a close just before shift change was about to happen when a bed alarm (an alarm that sounds when someone tries to get out of bed that isn't supposed to) went off. Someone shouted the room number and I thought 'that can't be.' It was my little volcano down the hall, but he never even attempts to get out of bed and he knows he is not supposed to. You never know what you will get when you rush in to take care of a bed alarm. I scurried over the long hallway to see if he had dropped something and leaned over or turned the wrong way when "bam" I heard a crash coming from his room. My quick step turned into a sprint and there he was in all his glory. It turns out I couldn't get a bed extender because he already had one. He stood about 8 feet tall, swaying and stumbling around the room. He had way too many opiate cocktails to be out of bed safely. I tried my best to get behind him and started to fuss. "What are you doing," I screeched. Part of it was surprise and shock at how ginormous he was and part was that they didn't teach us about keeping an unsteady giant from falling. I mean it was seriously like a Chihuahua trying to catch a Great-Dane. His rear end was literally bent over in my face and uncovered because of the doll-sized gown that left nothing to the imagination. "I need to use the bathroom," he said. I tried to get him to use the urinal like we had all weekend and he said, "What I have to do won't fit in there." I could say nothing but, "Oh." We scrambled around the room towards the bathroom as he swayed back and forth on his quivering, unsteady leg like a giant tree in a large hurricane that's about to plow over. We just about made it to the toilet seat when I tried to turn on the lights, but he said he didn't have enough time for that and smooshed me out the way. What could I do? I was ass to face with this guy, there's no arguing with that. He plopped down when I heard what seemed to be a bone hitting metal sound, "pop." That gentle giant turned into a grizzly giant shouting at the top of his lungs "Rape… rape!" He unknowingly hit the long retractable cleaning spigot on the commode that wasn't placed back properly after the last person cleaned out his urinal. He thought I tried to impale him with something because it was dark and he couldn't see. By this time, it is shift change so people from two shifts are piling in to see the spectacle of me trying to comfort what looked to be the stars, the sun and the moon because this guy was all exposed and that was the only view I had with him bent over in pain. He finally figured out I wasn't trying to rape him but determined I would kill him as he shouted, "She's killing me, she's killing me, I'm going to die." What do you even say to that? Let's just say that was a hard one to explain to my supervisor in writing.

MY APOLOGIES IF I OFFEND YOU

I feel awful for saying this, but I've noticed that most hard-core drug addicts are so resilient. They survive in the worst of the worst wrecks and thrive with taking in as much pain medicine as you can give. They have adapted to harsh environments in the outside world. I have given enough medicine to one individual that would put down an entire zoo. Crackheads are like cockroaches, no matter what you do to them they never die.

HOLES: EVERYBODY'S GOT ONE, RIGHT?

I finished my tasks fairly early one night and noticed a newer nurse with the look. You know the one, the deer in headlights look. I've been nursing for some time and am always glad to give a helping hand and drop some knowledge. She tells me she was trying to place a catheter and was having no luck. There were more words, but I didn't quite understand what she was saying. All I knew was that a catheter needed to be placed. She had the supplies ready to go and several other used materials that needed to be discarded. I tossed the trash while wondering what in the world is wrong with this girl that she can't place a catheter on this guy. I thought never mind that, I just went to business preparing and told the patient what I was doing. I gloved up, grabbed his inner leg and brought the tip of the catheter to his tip when I realized something very important. I looked high, I looked low. I couldn't find the hole. What the hell? I know everyone's anatomy is different, but this was not right. He must have peed somehow in his lifetime. I threw in the towel after about fifteen very confusing minutes but with my head still hung high until I came across the only two nurses available. The schedule just so worked out that both of the two highest supervisors were working and were the only ones with the knowledge and ability to help. I came to them with my legitimate problem and naturally was laughed at straight to my face, but they didn't have to point. They grabbed more supplies and were again faced with the problem of discovering where the hole could be. We sifted through the extra skin. We poked and prodded. Finally, someone had the bright idea to grab some numbing lube to make it easier for the patient. We squirted some on a new catheter and some straight into a crevice of skin where we suspected it could be tucked away on the bottom. As I squirted it in, a mound of puss sprayed out. I could feel pressure free up in my hand and was then able to place the catheter with minimal difficulty; but I have been catheter shy ever since, tucking my tail and cowering away at the thought of a cath.

ANGEL

I've known many people that have worn a halo (a birdcage-like metal contraption attached to the head and chest that does not allow for any neck motions) have never been close to resembling an angel. One female with one kept making love to her bed rail. I finally had to shut the door when she left a dark red slick behind from her menstrual cycle.

Best order ever written:

PT is to be done every day unless patient is currently receiving chest compressions

CODES

I was walking by a patient room and noticed a woman in a gown slumped over the bed and blue. I always carry my sheet that has all the patients listed with their code statuses (stating whether they would like to be saved or not if their heart stops) on them. I checked and saw she was considered to be a full code. I rush into her room and check for a pulse. Nothing. Ok, I guess we're doing this thing was what I said in my mind. I started applying chest compressions and called out for help. The code team hooked up a monitor when the patient startled up from the dead and screams "get off me". She wasn't the only one shaken by that. I quickly obliged and jumped off of her. Suddenly her body went limp again and the heart monitor alarmed with a flat line. I soared back on her and was about six pumps in when she again rose from the dead, but this time she punched me in the face and exclaimed, "Didn't I tell you to get off of me?"

YOU GOT TO TAKE THE GOOD WITH THE BAD

The bad news is that I barged in on a male getting some head. The good news is that I was coming in to clean his catheter, but it was already sparkling!

BROKEN BONES AND SPIRITS

A man came in with multiple broken bones. He had been inappropriate with all the female staff for days, so naturally, I was on high alert and guarded towards him. Not that I treated him any differently than any other person, I was just on my best behavior trying to keep it strictly professional so he didn't catch me off guard. It was my first time in his room and I had my back turned towards him as I was washing my hands to get started. He told me I was hot and that he needed someone hot like me to give him a bath. Out of nowhere I snapped at him and said, "Your hands aren't broken." Oh, but they were and boy was my face red! That was the first and last time my patient ever had to suffer at my expense from my word vomit.

THE BLUE WAFFLE

A male was settling into his hospital room after a bad sledding injury he endured. He looked healthy and wanted to get some rest; so I tried to make his admission history paperwork short, sweet and to the point. I asked him a few specific questions but then with the generalized inquiries I summed it up and asked, "Have you had or have you ever had any health problems?" He calmly said, "I have the blue waffle." I looked at him not comprehending thinking I missed something. After a brief staring competition, I gave in and asked, "what is a blue waffle. He looked disgusted and exclaimed, "You're a registered nurse and you don't know what the blue waffle is?" No, I had no clue of what this thing was. Google it, I dare you. I know my co-workers and I did and every computer for at least a month had those images in the background until the nurse educator discovered what it was. I tell you what, none of us knew what the blue waffle was that night, but none of us would ever forget it from here on out.

THINGS NOT TO DO

I have a list going of things not to do that my patients have done:

Cow tipping

Using a chainsaw over the age of 85 in a tree

Replacing a loose roof above the age of 90

Fall asleep on train tracks

Jump out of a car on the interstate for $1

Sledding off a mountain with cliffs in the summertime

Smack an angry person that has a gun

Bull riding

Russian roulette

Become a beekeeper with a bee allergy without proper equipment

Noodling aka "Redneck catfishing" where you use your arm or hand as bait (believe me it's not pretty)

Chasing someone with a firework

Jumping out and scaring people in a clown costume

CAUGHT WHITE-HANDED

A man came in because of a bad motorcycle accident. He had significant belly issues to be attended to while he was in the ICU. It had been several weeks before he got to join me on the step-down unit, but he finally did. He had hair for days and was obsessed with it. From the look of it, it was down the middle of his back. He tells me it generally goes past his buttocks and he would let none of those "banshees" touch his hair on the other floor. His hair had not been brushed during his entire hospital stay and he felt like he was doing me a favor by allowing me the honor of getting the tangles out. We were way beyond knots, tangles, and kinks; we were dealing with one single huge dreadlock. It was awful and the smell was horrendous. I rallied up the troops and instead of taking breaks, all the staff would come in with any of their own personal free time they had and try to tame the beast he called hair. If any of us even mentioned taking scissors to it, he would kick us out permanently. We did everything that we could for his hair and found all the products we could to make it easier, but it didn't do much use. A few days into this thing he got so fixated on it that he was on the brink of insanity for him. He tried everything he could and spent all his time combing and brushing. We had up to five people at times working on his scalp, but it still wasn't good enough. This had been ongoing for almost a week, I had to finally take a break and eat. When I came back he was covered with a white substance. It was the butt paste I use to batter up bottoms like a big old wedding cake that hardens. It was in his mouth, it was in his hair, it was in his crotch, it was everywhere. The fairly large tube started off brand new/full/unopened and was now empty. "I was using olive oil. What makes you think that butt paste was going to do the trick?" He didn't pick the smooth clear one, he went for the one that is like old-school toothpaste. As I'm assessing to see how bad the damage was, he grabbed my forearm which left a huge distinct hand imprint. I pulled away saying "No, I know where those hands have been," as I can see he clearly took a break when I did but he masturbated with his time. So he's sitting there explaining himself which didn't matter at this point because the damage was already done. I just wanted to know one thing, so I asked. "Why were you eating it?" He just stared at me stunned that I called him out. I exited the room to wash the caked-on crust off of my arm. I was double digits deep in the number of times that it took to wash that man-juice paste off and it was still there! And everyone was questioning what was wrong with my arm and I would just simply say, "You know, curiosity killed the cat," as I would walk off repulsed and embarrassed having to relive the moment. Once I regrouped and forced myself back into his room, he told me to cut his hair. I figured that he had a moment of clarity or maybe he put himself in our shoes. I didn't waste time questioning it just in case he changed his mind, so I grabbed the pair in my pocket and cut the one very large troublesome knot trying to sift my way through consolidating as little collateral damage as possible. He snatched the wad of knotted hair and went to work on it. I asked him what he was doing, and he said, "Oh you'll see." Later, I came back and there was what looked to be a doll in his hand as he slept. I said to myself, 'Aww, how cute.' He spontaneously opened his eyes and looked at me and said, "You won't think it's cute when it brings you great harm. You don't recognize it?" he asked. I shook my head no in disbelief. He continued on, "This is my nurse Voodoo Doll. I'm going to bring harm to all those that caused me to go bald." He then stuck it in his backpack and started to chant some language that I'm pretty sure he made up and meditated. You would think he'd be a little more grateful with all the man hours we put into his man-do! I think twice before helping anyone now.

SELFISH

I had taken care of a gentleman with a bad injury from a fall and had to have multiple surgeries. He had been living alone for years after his wife passed and had gotten to where he was barely functional. I do not understand how he survived at the level he was at. He was very confused, couldn't feed himself or even make decisions for himself. He must have been multiple falls for a long time because he had many bumps and bruises all over his body. We tracked down his daughter and she stopped by. She didn't seem troubled with how he was doing and didn't realize how bad off he was cognitively. She was mostly concerned about the hospital bill falling on her and how much it would cost to place him in a permanent living facility. She left and didn't visit again. Weeks later I received a call from her to check up on her dad. I recognized her voice and thought that she was so cold towards him before and hoped that she would get involved more. I answered her questions and let her know what was going on with him and his care. Later that day, I was pulled off the floor into the Nurse Manager's office. It's the worst feeling in the world to be summoned like that. It's like you are in high school all over again being paged overhead to go to the principal's office. Generally, it's not for anything good and everyone knows that you are in there. My manager told me she got a call earlier that day from my patient's daughter. She says that she was highly upset and offended that I would just readily give her father's personal information out. She wanted me terminated and my nursing license removed. What kind of shit is this? I took very good care of her dad. I caught that he had a large bleed that he had to go straight for an emergent surgery for which probably saved his life. Not everyone looks at the lab levels and the vital sign trends the way that I analyze them, which is how I figured out that something was wrong that everyone else had missed because good nurses do that. I was immediately suspended pending an investigation. The daughter had been so gracious to record our conversation so she could have evidence against me and was threatening to sue the hospital, stating that if I was so willing to give out information to her so easily without her being his official Medical POA (Power of Attorney-a designated person that makes decisions about a person's medical care), then who else would I give information to? In my state, when a person is deemed incompetent and cannot make their own decisions if they do not have paperwork for a POA, then your closest next of kin can make decisions. In my patient's case, his daughter could not be contacted initially, so all of his consents were signed by two doctors for him to get the care he needed until a family member was found. I had met her in person in the room and knew her voice, so I saw no problem including her in his care since there is a huge push to do so because it is a basis of patient-centered care. I broke no laws and felt I had the patient's best interests at heart the entire time. During the investigation, the daughter had a meeting with one of the elite personnel that aids to protect the best interests of the hospital. In that meeting, she said she would not pursue a lawsuit if the hospital removed her father's bill and found him a place to reside that would cost no money out of pocket. But she had to stick to her guns so as part of her bargaining chip she wanted my license to be revoked. As I understand it, there was some back and forth and ultimately that day her father's hospital bill disappeared along with my job. Her end game all along was all about money; no one can convince me otherwise. I'm not too sure if she was compensated for the pain and suffering she claimed to endure in this process but at least I salvaged my license.

THE FOREVER FORGOTTEN

I went to help a patient clean himself that had urinated. He could not assist because of his injury. As I began, he exclaims, "Sorry if I get one, sorry if I don't." Doesn't he know that we look but we don't see? As in, we see what we need to and it is forgotten shortly afterward for both of our sakes.

EVERYBODY'S GOT A DREAM

I love sending the biggest, burliest, hairiest man I can find to give a bed bath or do a catheter insertion when they request the sexiest nurse to do it. I'm sure that nurse is sexy to someone, just not that patient. I don't know if that patient enjoys it, but I do.

DESPERATION

I had a guy that was so hard up in his addiction he had been cheeking (hiding medications between the inner cheek and outer teeth) his oxycodone and using a flush (used hospital syringe) he found to administer his poop-juice water left in his bedpan. He had to remain in the hospital for an extended amount of time for a major bloodstream infection.

DISCHARGED FOR ETERNITY

I was discharging a patient medically cleared to leave. All of her tubes had been removed and she was in her regular street clothes. I reviewed the discharge instructions with her and her husband and then sent him out to the car with her belongings to pick her up at the discharge area, but almost as soon as he left, the patient collapsed on the bed. She was not breathing and there was no pulse. I called a code blue and we worked hard to bring her back. She had no IV access to administer any lifesaving medications and we were not capable of accurately placing one due to blood not flowing through on its own and the movement from the CPR made it impossible. Eventually we placed a central line (similar to an IV but it is placed in larger vessels) but unfortunately, it was too little, too late. She was dead. Meanwhile, her husband of fifty years the next month grew weary of waiting and headed back towards the unit. One of our staff members seemed a little caught up in the moment and decided it was a good idea to greet him at the elevators just outside of the unit and let him know in a matter of fact way stating, "She's dead." That's it, "She's dead," was all that was said. No graceful introduction, compassion or empathy. Now before anyone is discharged, taking an IV out is always the last thing I ever do because I still hear his bloodcurdling screams in my mind to this day.

GOT SALAD?

You ever notice that people that speak a foreign language have an accent that seems to go away when they sing in English no matter how thick their accent is? It's kind of like when you piss off a patient with word salad (a brain issue that mixes up the words a person is trying to get out, making communication very difficult and frustrating). It's like the moment they get angry and turn into the Hulk or Hulk-tress and cuss you out for everything you are worth; but their speech morphs from improperly put together sentences to beautifully articulated, streamlined ones that make perfect sense.

STIFF

I was walking down the hallway at the end of my shift and noticed a very off color of a patient. She didn't look right. I figured I would check on her since it's not like her nurse would get off her tail to lay eyes on her. Upon further investigation, she was completely blue and motionless. There was no DNR (do not resuscitate) armband, so I immediately called a code blue (an alarm for immediate assistance for someone whose heart or breathing stopped). The bed was in an upright position, so I used the CPR button to flatten it out in an instance. The bed flattened, but she did not. Her back went down and her legs and feet went straight up. She was so past dead, she was in full on rigger! The hospital policy stated that a patient was not deemed deceased until a medical doctor examines the patient, determines that the heart is not beating and calls an official time of death so we had to work the code as if that person had a fighting chance. Do you know how hard and awkward it is to get on someone's chest and do compressions while their legs and feet are straight in the air?

DRIVING WHILE INEBRIATED

A man came into the hospital pretty broken up. He had multiple broken bones including his back, ribs, arms, and legs. He appeared to be highly inebriated. Whatever he was on he was sleeping off as it didn't show up on his toxicology screen. He needed his rest because come morning he would be arrested. It's a big deal to be arrested while hospitalized as the county must pay for all charges incurred during that visit. Whatever he did must have been awful for the county to do that as opposed to waiting till being discharged and not having a bill. When a person is arrested while in the hospital, usually, the county is just trying to please the public. Come to find out when reading the warrant on his chart, I saw just what the charges were for, and that information is not always on the write-up in the chart. While speeding in the wrong lane he hit another vehicle head-on. That vehicle contained a family of five; a father, a mother, twin toddlers and an infant coming back from vacationing. All dead! He had no idea what he had done. In the morning, as planned he was arrested. His world came crashing down and the dead family's surviving members worlds were shattered. He was devastated. How could he have done such a thing? He had never even had so much as a drop of alcohol or a traffic violation in his life. He had recently changed doctors. In that transition, he told his new doctor the four medications he was taking. They prescribed him four medications. He took the medications following the directions to the letter on the bottles. Upon further investigation, it turns out that he was originally prescribed the four medications in the brand name, then prescribed the exact same medications, but the generic versions to save on cost (the initial reason for changing doctors). He was essentially taking double his prescribed medications, all of which were mind-altering when consumed in high doses. He killed five people, injured himself badly and had no memory of it. Even though he would not have done this without the prescribed medicines, he still held himself accountable because he felt that if it weren't for him that family would still be alive. Now someone else gets to read his son a story every night as he remains on suicide watch because he won't get to do this for several decades.

Students

There is a special place in my heart for students. They are like fresh sponges ready to be absorbed that haven't been tainted yet. This one is for the students...

YEASTY BEASTY

A few students were in a patient's room with me learning how to properly place a catheter. There was an odor when separating the patient's legs. The way I figure is that it doesn't matter what's on the outside as long as you get what's on the inside...liquid gold. One student leaned back. I pushed him forward and gave him a look. He straightened up and we got back to business. As we were finishing up, I showed them a skin moisture issue that appeared to be rampant down there, so they know what to look for if they ever saw it again. I pointed it out and said it could be yeast. This is when a different student came up, reached his hand down there to graze the affected area and brought it up to his nose and said, "It doesn't smell like yeast."

BEST PATIENT QUOTES OF ALL TIMES

"Yeah, well, your mom had an ugly daughter" (patient) "Oh, I see you met my sister" (my response)

"I'm going to trade my beer cap in for a 90-day chip"

"I can't wear that gown, there's no dick hole in it"

"You may be strong, but odor isn't everything"

"Who you got to deep throat around here to get your glasses fixed" (hours later with the same patent...)

"I'd deep throat somebody for a pair of glasses right about now"

"No, no, I'm not going to kill them... yet" (talking to his invisible friend about the staff)

"I do retox not detox"

"I'm in between sobriety"

"If he's got the balls, tell him to bring them to me"

"If I was a dog, I wouldn't get in as much trouble because if I could lick myself like them, I'd never leave the house"

"If I could get out this contraption of a bed I'd kick his ass"

"I'm not wearing that dress (gown); it doesn't have a dick hole in it"

"I guess you're the boss because you're wearing the pants and I'm wearing the dress"

"Now I won't hit a woman, but I'll smack a bitch"

VANITY

I was having a good run of luck during my shift where all my patients were sleeping. I got all of my tasks accomplished so I asked around to see if anyone needed anything. There was a patient that was one-to-one, where someone had to sit with her at all times for safety. That person's female sitter called out consistently for numerous breaks and I was the only person that had not relieved her yet. I am a male nurse and I prefer not to go into female patient rooms, so the other collogues were relieving her. The sitter called out yet again for another break but there was no one that could go, so it was my turn. As I approached the door, the sitter darted out like she was going to mess herself. I didn't think much of it. I grazed in and the patient was lying on the bed quietly. When she saw me, she quickly sat up on the side of the bed and watched me watch her. After about a minute of the creepiest stare down of my life, she pats the bed and asks me to sit with her. No was not an acceptable answer to her. She kept pawing at the bed and harassing me to come closer. She then slithered off the bed to crawl towards me. I assisted her to get off the floor and she was grabbing at my junk. This is not good. A woman's scorn can run deep with a man telling her no. She could make up a story and tell people anything she wants to which can cause a nurse to get fired or lose their license. I called out and pleaded for someone to come relieve me, but no one came. Finally, the sitter came back to relieve me. The fifteen minutes she took felt like an eternity. I was already at the door itching to get out, but I needed to tell her what went on so I would have someone knowing I'm not trying to change up the story of what went down in there. I frantically told her what happened when she cut me off and exclaimed, "You're not special. She does that same thing to me and everyone else that walks through this door." Suddenly I just felt used like the gum at the bottom of someone's shoe.

NAKED AND AFRAID

There was a man we nursing staff called Angry Santa. He looked just like you would imagine a real-life Santa Claus would; so kind, sweet and jolly but looks are deceiving. He was generally yelling, slapping, kicking, spitting and taking his clothes off. Now I am quick to tie someone up like a little pig if they become violent. Nothing is like having a little nurse abuse to start your day. I had to restrain him straight from the beginning of my shift; both hands and feet but also a mask to prevent him from spitting in my face again. With his continuous baseline anger, he would have an occasional bout of kindness that would shine through occasionally. He needed to use the bathroom in a hurry and I couldn't find any help. Against my better judgment, I unhooked him and allowed him to walk to get his poop on in the nude. He handled his business and didn't want to go back to bed. His anger revived again as he pulled on my shirt. He was a big guy with a ginormous amount of strength. He kept tugging to get away from the bed and I kept squirming towards it until it happened. He was holding my shirt in his hands and trying to fight me. I like to think of myself as half man and half amazing but standing there half naked trying to protect a naked man from himself, I determined was not a good look. You can ask for help, but a nurse always knows it may come, but at a price. Decisions! At what point does modesty hinder safety? Well, I discovered that day when I was throat-popped avoiding a strong unsteady fist as opposed to the wrath I would've felt from my coworkers for months. Some wounds don't heal, I figured I could get over a sore throat but I'd never get away from the memory this would leave behind. With all the commotion going on, my worst fear happened anyway. The Calvary came in to save me. There I was being chased half-naked by a very unsteady Naked Naughty Santa. It's like the image was burned into their retinas.

DON'T BITE THE HAND

A man was admitted for some serious belly issues. He was an interesting character and I enjoyed my time with him telling me interesting stories of what he had to do to pay for his illegal habits (like dress up as a woman and solicit himself, which never seemed to turn out the way he thought it would) and some of the crazy things his friends would do when they were inebriated (such as inconspicuously pooping in the crack of a doorway so the next person walking in would step into it). Don't be fooled; he was fun to joke with but was the opposite end of that spectrum when I was on his shit list for something the doctor ordered that I had no control over. It was on. I will just say you don't want to be the one that pisses off someone that shits on their friend's floor for giggles. Suddenly I was the worst person in the world to him and he let that be known by doing little things to annoy me. For instance, he used his flat sheet to tie one end onto the door handle and the other created a noose around his neck; so when anyone came into his room he pretended to be dead. He would also lie down on the floor and pretend he fell. Oh, I forgot to mention he had only one leg. Due to his misbehavior and physical ailment he had to have a chair alarm to prevent him from falling, so that every time he stood up the alarm would go off. Just for fun, he would stand to let the alarm beep so I would have to run and right before I entered he would sit back on it to make it stop. He was so good at this that he listened for the specific sound of my voice and footsteps. It's amazing what people will drum up with enough time and willpower. He didn't feel like he was getting enough pain medicine which prompted all this aggression towards me. The doctors felt like he was abusing his as-needed pain medicine so they were tapering him down to get him off of them. He had been on them for years and had an acute (new) injury and now the doctors were speaking with his pain management doctors to get him off them permanently. The only thing that made his day worthwhile was to make sure that I earned my keep. Well, we played this reindeer game for two days in a row, until I found him passed out in the chair with his prosthetic leg in the floor and an open secret hidden compartment full of a junkie's dream he had been using since he had been there. He was then stripped of his chair privilege and was given a medication to reverse what he had taken. This is the one thing that a true addict can't stand; you can literally bring them back from the dead with this medicine and they are furious because you ruined their high. It's like swinging a stick blindfolded at a beehive as if it were a piñata because you should expect retaliation. At this point, he was kicking and screaming. His little nub was going to town as he threatened to kick me with it. I was about at the end of my rope with this guy who had abused my patience for days, so I simply told him, "You know, you don't bite the hand that feeds you pain medicine. I'm going to let you chew on that for a few minutes and come back." I then left the room, came back a few minutes later and we were friends again. I left that day with my head held high thinking what a good job I did. I set that next nurse up for success. But that success came crashing down into disaster when I came back for my next shift and saw her typing with a bloodied wrap around her hand. Apparently, this guy took my statement to heart when he discovered that his secret stash had been removed and disposed of. He then threw a fit, punched one nurse in the face and bit the hand of the one I gave a report to (who by the way just discovered she was pregnant during that shift when she wasn't supposed to have any more children because pregnancy was so rough for her). Who needs enemies when you have friends like this guy?

GREEN

I was asked to help out in a room that had just called out and requested a catheter to be brought. I knew what time it was; it was time for me to show off how good I am at placing a difficult catheter. So I strutted in the room guns blazing ready to seal the deal with this catheter. Now I've been a nurse for a long time and it takes a lot to impress me and a lot to make me do a double take at something out of the ordinary. The catheter was not a problem and was easy to get in. The staff working with the patient just wanted to see my face when I went to place the catheter. No kidding. It was so big that I had to get a special catheter called a Foley instead of the Red Robinson I would normally use for an in and out because it could not reach his bladder. That's impressive and I don't say that often about anything. All the male nurses that week were walking around butt-hurt and appeared to suffer from a mad case of penis envy, saying things like, "Oh, he's just a shower, not a grower." I can assure you he was more than just a shower, but a grower as well as he enjoyed getting the catheter. He enjoyed it so much that if sometimes when the catheter was removed after emptying his bladder, something other than urine would follow.

Best Tattoos:

"Your name"

Mustache on finger (which brought a whole new meaning to finger mustache)

Tweety bird mowing (around the groin area)

Suffering succotash waxing (in-between the groin areas)

"DNR" on chest

An air balloon coming out of someone's rear end that said "hot air"

The word "Luscious" could be visualized when you pulled apart a certain set of fat rolls

"Dr. Knee Knocker"

"Drive like Hell and you'll get there"

"Slug Life" was misspelled on his back instead of Thug Life (because the person had a very large lisp)

"Do not remove above a perforated line" around a patient's only leg with a perforated line mark

A cat that appeared to lick their nipple

Read between the lines as a tramp stamp on an older woman with another one that said lick when separating her buttocks

EVERYBODY DOES IT

I give every patient the opportunity to try to poop on their own accord. There comes a point where I must take over and give a helping hand. Generally, that is when a patient looks to be about 8 months pregnant, but they are a male in their 80s. This is a real thing that can happen and cause significant harm, including death. There is only so much you can pack in your body before there are irreversible problems. When I intervene, I try to start at the front door and if that doesn't work I go to the back door. I had a patient that went over a week without having a bowel movement. Some people say this is typical and they are out there, but I don't care because it's not supposed to be normal. Everyone is different, but it is not typical to go more than a week without pooping, especially in the trauma setting. They don't call me the Poo Queen for nothing. I am an advocate for it. I make sure all my folks go. One day I had a patient that went ten days without going and was getting very uncomfortable. I kept asking if she felt anything at her backdoor and the answer was always "no." I tried everything that I could think of before having to go the enema route. It was my last resort and we were there. I collected my equipment and set up shop. I was on one side of the bed and I had two other nurses on the other to help with comfort and positioning as this is best to do with an injured patient in a side-lying position. I got the entire bag of enema medicine inserted and waited a few minutes for the magic to happen. When suddenly she quivered and hastily blurts out, "It's tapping at my back door now." I could literally hear it brewing inside of her. It was about to hit, and it was about to hit hard. I had a choice to make. It's like there was an Angel on the right shoulder saying, "Don't do it" and a Devil on the other saying, "Point that thing over there." Oh, the choices. I should feel bad because I did not take the high road. I was the main nurse who knows the ailments of the patient, so it was my responsibility to turn the patient in the appropriate direction. I did bad. I turned her onto her broken hip without thinking and just as soon as I did there was a horrendous noise that sounded like a giant firecracker going off. Feces went flying in all directions like shrapnel from a bomb explosion. Crap was literally all over the nurses. It even went inside one of their mouths and was dripping from her lip. They were troopers and toughed it out until the end. That's what being a nurse is about; you never let them see you sweat. But that doesn't mean you can't ignore someone because to this day that nurse still won't talk to me. I try to reassure her to the best of my abilities and tell her that it's ok because she has a shitty mouth anyways.

NO WORDS

A man came in very confused after being assaulted in a parking lot. He initially arrived at his room straight after surgery and could not answer questions. I did my best to do a thorough skin assessment on him but was incapable of seeing his entire backside as he weighed almost a thousand pounds. We did not have the proper equipment or staffing to accommodate this. I just made sure to squirrel in as many pillows as I could under him every two hours, plus alternate which side of him to place the pillows to prevent any pressure ulcers. He was very needy. He wanted someone in the room at all times. He generally used the call-bell to ask for assistance about ninety times for each twelve-hour shift. As soon as each staff member left the room, he would call them to come directly back. Once after being caught up in his room for an hour, I went to attend to my other patients. I could hear him yelling out to the patient across the hall. He had that person chant "help" in sequence simultaneously for fifteen minutes till someone came in. He just wanted someone to fluff his pillow and scratch his back and chest. Something he could have done himself, mind you. As the weeks passed, he got better; still needy, but the confusion dissipated. Since he was lucid I had to get his medication list and a medical history. Beyond the obvious morbid obesity, he was healthy except for one thing. He said that he was using a cream for something that he couldn't put his finger on for some skin issue. I did some digging and come to find out he had scabies. Holly hell! Of all things to have, he had to have scabies. It's itchy and highly contagious. He had been there for weeks and everyone that worked there and then some came into his room and touched on him somehow, some way. We all wash our hands when we go in and come out of all rooms, but just the thought of it made us itch for days thinking we had something.

WASTED EFFORTS

A lady came into the Emergency Room demanding to get a particular high-grade IV pain medicine. There was no real indication for her to receive it, so her ten-hour wait in the Emergency Room was worthless. She was quickly sent on her merry way empty-handed. She wanted this IV medicine so badly that when she exited the hospital, she marched straight into the nearest grocery store and stabbed herself to create a reason for it. Since she went to such extreme measures to acquire this medicine, we basically viewed it as an allergy because if she would stab herself to get a dose or two, what would she do for more? Try not to think of us as cruel, but if a sane person actually tries to stab themselves, it is hard to hit anything vital because our brain tries to force our body to stop because the pain is so intense. Because of this, her wounds were mostly superficial. She went through all that trouble for only some Ibuprofen and IV Tylenol.

CHOOSE YOUR BATTLES WISELY

Some events arise occasionally that, as nurses, we must take one for the team. Most of the time you don't know it's about to happen until you are there in it. It's basically like when you step in fresh dog poo, you are already there and there's no going back. Sometimes you just have to close your eyes and go with it. For example: let's say there is a nervous, confused patient who needs a large dressing change. You bring an extra set of hands or two for moral support and to hold the patient in place, but as a distraction, the patient begins to feel on your booty. What do you do when he doesn't listen? Do you stop the painful procedure and take your clean gloves off to remove his hand when it will just add time you don't have, plus his hand will go right back, or do you roll with plan B and go with it? Ding, ding, ding… plan B is correct. It's not about you. It's about what's best for the patient. You just continue on with what you are doing and pretend you are at the club where you know an ugly person has come up behind you and is breathing on your neck, but you don't turn around because you already know what's on the other side. Either way, let's be real; for most nurses, it's probably the most action you will see in a month. I guess inappropriate touch Tuesday sometimes turns into Molestation Monday.

THE CRAIGSLIST GEM

A very robust female came in with a stab wound to her arm from a stiletto heel. You don't have that kind of wound without some drama behind it. Better yet, it was the second time she was stabbed in one week; two separate events, but who am I to judge? It's not my place to form a predisposed opinion about anyone. It doesn't matter what patients have done, only how we can affect their present and future in a positive light. She was in the middle of a very long road with us and was "so bored," all she wanted to do was get out the hospital. When you have been through a traumatic event, looked death square in the face and lived to tell about it, your perception generally changes. When you get out of the hospital, it's like the sky is bluer, the grass is greener and things taste better. She just wanted a taste of freedom, but that was against policy as she had a device on her arm called a wound VAC to allow her to heal faster and prevent infection. She was so frustrated in her hospital-acquired purgatory she snuck out. Nothing like going home and telling your spouse, 'Hey honey, I lost a patient today, I hope they went to a better place.' When she eventually came back, I fussed at her, "Do you realize how nobody comes here when they are feeling good?" She didn't care. She continued to sneak out and was making a habit of it. We wondered what she was up to. It's not like there were tons of things to do around the hospital. One day a man came up to the desk asking for her by her nickname. He didn't look like he knew her. He went to her room and she sent him out. I thought it was fishy and I had a few minutes, so I waited and caught her trying to creep out, but this time, I let her and I followed. She went out to the parking lot and into the visiting man's car. It didn't take long for it to start rocking and I wasn't about to start knocking. I went back up knowing it wouldn't be long before she would come tiptoeing back to her room. When she came back, I confronted her. She admitted that she had been posting ads on Craigslist to do favors to get some vending machine money for moon pies and RC colas. We kept telling her how unsafe it was to play with strangers, but she kept doing what it took to get her candy cash. She continued doing this for a few weeks until one day it miraculously stopped without us having to intervene. Sometimes you just must give thanks for the little things.

TWO BIRDS, ONE STONE

A horrific smell was seeping down the hallway and into the nurses' station. At first, it would graze by and be gone. Then, it was a faint linger in the background and after about a week it was prominently throughout the hallway, where when you went home you brought the smell with you because it was in your clothes. We searched high and low, top to bottom as the odor had made it into four patient rooms. The pungent aroma finally got to a point we could tell distinctly which room it belonged to, but still couldn't pinpoint it. Finally, the girl menstruated and when she went to remove her tampon, two came out instead of one. It had been in there for an entire month, but it took over three for the smell to go away. This patient was none other than our very own Craigslist Gem.

THE UGLY

NEVER AGAIN

A patient needed an NG (Nasogastric tube – a tube that goes from the nose straight to the stomach that can remove or administer fluids). I am an old-school nurse with many tricks up my sleeve. I used one of my tricks that I always do for this. I placed the sealed, double packaged tube in a bag of ice and put it in the refrigerator for a while. It stiffens it up to allow for easy placement. I placed the tube with no complications as always, checked it myself and then verified it with another nurse using the auscultation method (listening via stethoscope). Later that night well after the tube was placed; the patient had trouble breathing and had to go to the ICU (Intensive Care Unit-where the sickest of the sick people go). The patient's stomach had been perforated. I heard she had a nice funeral.

THE ONE-HANDED HIGH-FIVE

A very large group came to visit a patient on the unit while I was in the room. They came bearing great news. They had raised $18,000 from a huge fundraiser they had been doing for a long period with many man hours of work. The benefit was for him, to aid in the treatment for his cancer. Everyone was so happy and proud including the patient. It was written all over their faces. High-fives and handshakes were going on all around. I wonder what they would have said if I told them he has never had cancer. He had to have multiple surgeries because he got too many live hamsters that died trying to get out his back door. When it was my turn to share the triumph, that was one high-five I had to leave hanging.

GOD VS. VANITY – NINE LIVES

Newlyweds were out celebrating. The woman was driving, and the man was popping out the sunroof like a jack in the box. Along came a sharp curve with an 18-wheeler behind it on the opposite side of the road. The two vehicles collided, and the impact sent the young man flying out the vehicle headfirst and straight into the bumper of the 18-wheeler. He seemed to break a little bit of everything and the only thing that saved his life was that he essentially was given a craniotomy (an opening into the skull to allow for swelling without compressing the brain) when his head hit during the crash; unfortunately, he could not get adequate blood flow to his brain to allow for any future brain function. His wife was also placed in the hospital but was now (by law) his Power of Attorney and had to make all decisions for herself and for him. Neither of them had anyone but each other. No friends, no family, no one. They were the lone rangers and liked it that way. Being alone and single was new to her and so was making tough decisions by herself; especially all while being injured, stressed and in pain. Some people came into her hospital room to talk to her about organ donation which made her feel better if there was any silver lining to the whole situation. She set a time for the plug to be pulled so she could coordinate a time and ensure that she would be there for a few minutes with her longtime love before he passed. Meanwhile, she tried to seek comfort the best way she could so she reached out. She called a nearby church and members came by to comfort her. They went above and beyond to console her by listening to her story and were moved. They were so moved, they prayed. They concluded that the doctors were wrong. They promised her that power of prayer could and would heal her wounded husband. She then drank the metaphorical kool-aid and went with it. They made a huge promise to bring back the only thing she wanted in this world, her husband by praying. The thing is that we could see from scanning him he wasn't getting any necessary blood to his brain which renders you brain-dead. It's like having a beautiful, flourishing flower that thrived but one day you stopped watering it. It needs water to survive, so without the water, it dies and you can't reverse dying. There's no turning back, what's dead is dead. No matter what you do to that flower after it withered away without water will not bring it back. Same as the brain, once it goes too long without oxygen (which blood carries) it dies, and you can't cure death. He endured multiple surgeries; painful surgeries not only on his head and face but his arms, legs, hips, back, and abdomen. Months after months went by with no improvement. He was deteriorating and his body could not even regulate its own temperature. The church members dropped off one by one until one day they did not stop by any more or even pick up the phone when she called. She was now released from the hospital and alone yet again but this time she was at the bedside of her love watching him decline and suffer day in and day out. She started to drink. She would go for short breaks out of the room and stumble back in reeking of alcohol. She still held her ground and believed he would get better. She had come too far just to let him go. So every time his heart stopped we would have to perform CPR to bring his body back. We broke each of his ribs in multiple places on multiple occasions. This went on and on until one day there was no coming back for him. His heart finally gave out. They were on the road to a debt-free life. Before the accident, they lived meagerly. They lived in a small house they bought together and worked numerous hours above the standard forty every week so one day they could have kids, take vacations and just enjoy each other. Since her hospitalization, she could not work due to her injuries and could not for some time after that. Just because you are in the hospital does not mean that your bills stop. People do not think about these things. She had no income and still needed to eat. It didn't take her long to blow through their life savings they had built together. Now that she had no way of paying her regular bills and the hospital bills started to come for her and him, she could not pay. She lost her house to foreclosure and had to live on the street, as her car was totaled in the crash and the 18-wheeler's insurance was maxed out. She had no way of paying for a funeral and the church that was so quick to embrace her, refused to even hold a service for him. She could not claim his body because she had no means to put him in the ground, so the county was forced to pay for him to be cremated. The truly sad part is that since he could not regulate his temperatures he ran extraordinarily high fevers which rendered him an inappropriate candidate to donate his organs. The one thing that once comforted her now haunts her. That there was an actual list of nine people who were all prepping for surgery when the original date and time was set to harvest his organs. All nine lives would have been saved but in the end died without her husband's lifesaving body parts.

THE UNANSWERED CALL OF DOOM

A couple was on a casual outing enjoying each other's company on a stroll in their car. The passenger had his legs crossed and feet kicked up on the dashboard relaxing. Traffic got congested when the driver had to slam on the brakes because the car in front of him did. The car behind them could not brake fast enough and tapped their bumper from behind. No one had any notable injuries as it was nothing more than a low-speed tap. No damage was even done to either vehicle. The driver felt fine and went home to rest while the passenger was urged to take a ride in the ambulance because his blood pressure would not stay under control. Everything was going well until he stood to get up from the stretcher to walk to the hospital bed and collapsed. We immediately moved his limp body to the bed. He could feel nothing from his waist down. We did scan after scan and multiple tests. It was official; he was paralyzed. As this was happening, his blood pressure continued to plummet. "I won't live like this! I refuse to live like this," he yelled. With all the testing, the only true injury was to his spine. He was alert and oriented and ultimately able to legally make his own decisions about his care. He had the right to refuse and that he did. He refused all lifesaving care. We scrambled trying to call his husband but there was no answer. His body was in shock and we could do nothing about it. We could not bring the use of his legs back, so he rejected the medications to stabilize his blood pressure. Once his final decision was made, it only took a few minutes for him to pass but it felt like an eternity. I bet his husband will think twice before missing another phone call again.

KINDNESS GOES A LONG WAY

A young lady was in a terrible accident after recently losing her husband from a separate event that happened weeks prior that. The crash killed the driver and left her unable to speak, eat or have any fluid/meaningful body movements. She is now fed through a painful tube; her brain does not allow her to sleep for over 4 hours a day and she will spend the rest of her life in a nursing home from this wreck. Upon police investigation, they could find no link between the driver and the passenger. They eventually found out where she lived and did a search where they finally found their answer. On her pillow, there was a note she had written. In the note, she explained that she couldn't live without her husband and planned to die by hitchhiking on the interstate and turning the steering wheel down a certain steep embankment. Let me say this: in this field, you notice a few things. One very important realization is there are some fates worse than death. At least her family can visit her throughout her long, painful journey trapped in a body that doesn't move and unable to communicate but with a fully functional mind; but that's more than I can say for that kind Samaritan.

GLORY

A girl was continuously admitted to the hospital. She never felt good. Physically she looked ok, but her lab work was off. Something was not right but we could never figure out the problem. She would stay for a week or two, feel better, discharge and would be right back within the month. The last few times she came in she was looking and feeling worse than ever before. We still couldn't find the route of the problem. Her mom was very involved, concerned, intrusive, clingy and overbearing. She couldn't stand that we couldn't give her the answer to what was happening to her daughter. The patient became very sick and had to be sent to the ICU. Her organs were shutting down, so we were doing everything we could to prevent any further damage and to reverse what we could. In the process, she could not have most pain medicines because it would interact with the medicines that she was receiving. This did not fly well with her mother. She went off on us as if we were the reason that her daughter was sick and tried to force our hand to give her pain medicine. We kept trying to explain that you must solve the problem, not mask it. She didn't understand this concept but was there every day bashing us. It was to the point I couldn't take it anymore and told her that it's not about you, it's about your daughter and if you have a problem with that I get off at seven and you can meet me outside in the parking lot. She didn't fuss at me anymore after that but not too long after her daughter took a turn for the worse and died. It was a long investigation and her mom did not take it well. She placed blame on everyone but there was one doctor in particular she felt was especially liable. We did everything for this girl. There was truly nothing more we could have done to save her life. The mom continued to call the hospital and harass the staff and the doctor. She just lost her daughter, so we allowed it to go on. One day the mom couldn't get in touch with the doctor because she was in surgery. She couldn't take it anymore. She came into the hospital like she occasionally did and instead of waiting, barged into the surgery room during an operation in a vengeful rage and shot the doctor to death. Security was right behind her and apprehended her before she could fire off at anyone else. That's when I learned a hard lesson and I stopped telling people what time I get off even when they threaten my life. The kicker of this story is that the mother had no one else to blame but herself because come to find out the meds she was sneaking in and giving her daughter caused her to hemorrhage (bleed out). The autopsy also found that the girl had been continuously poisoned for years. The mom was so starved for attention she was making her daughter sick to get attention and the glory.

UNJUST

A lady was being sent from the ICU to the trauma unit just to die. Death was fast approaching, and she was not expected to live after being extubated (a tube to breaths for your body). They needed the room in the ICU and she would not make it through the night to be transferred to hospice. She suffered a massive gunshot wound to the head. The report given said that it was self-inflicted, and her husband heard it from the next room. She looked so sad lying there with only a bloodied gauze wrap around her swollen head. The room was cold. Her mind and body appeared to hold so many secrets. When looking at her CT scan there was a clear entry wound from the side/back part of her head. There was no plausible way she could have shot herself. When I called the Emergency Room for more clarity on her situation, there was something strange that was off when she came in. Her wound was barely bleeding and all the blood on her clothes was dried. This is not normal, especially when the husband said that he called 911 immediately and it took them only 17 minutes to collect her and bring her back since they lived so close. The husband did it and if he didn't, he was protecting the person that did. He didn't come to the hospital knowing she had only minutes to hours to live. He didn't even bother to call and check up on her. She had no friends and no family in the world. Her husband was the only person she had. She also had multiple wounds all over the trunk of her body in various stages of healing. She had been beaten for a long time in places that could not be seen with her clothes on. I called and reported my findings to everyone I could, but it was useless. Somehow the police said it was suicide and that was that. There was not even an investigation. Beyond not calling to check to see if her chest was rising and falling still, once she passed he wouldn't even claim her body. The city had to take over and cremate her remains. I stayed with her until she took her last breath and held her hand. That's the only gift I could give to her; the gift of compassion and togetherness. I swear the temperature of the room went up about 10 degrees as whatever was left inside of her left her body.

ONE IS THE LONELIEST NUMBER

There was a young lady who had been segregated from the world her entire life. Her parents had a phobia of people. She was homeschooled and the only friends she ever had were her immediate family members. She was very lonely and yearning for love. All she knew was that she wanted a baby so desperately she would do anything for it. Her parents wanted her to remain innocent and exiled her from other girls and boys alike. Her grandmother once told her that babies come from sewing a chicken breast inside of your uterus. It's amazing what people will do with enough willpower and time on their hands. Her yearning and desire got the best of her, so she went for it. She picked the best chicken from the coop on her family's land. When her parents fell asleep she cut off the chicken's head, plucked it and disassembled it, taking only the breast for herself. She cooked the rest of the chicken for her family because "that's what good mothers do." About a week went by, her belly started to "grow." She was so elated, but she didn't know how to tell her family she was going to have a child. They wouldn't think that she was ready; so, she decided to prove herself. She did extra chores around the house. She was also figuring out the best time to let her family know about the exciting news and how to tell them. A few days later there was a smell. At first, it would pass by every now and again. She chalked it up to an increased sense of smell from the pregnancy. At some point, her parents noticed the offensive aroma as well but she shrugged them off saying it was nothing. She became nauseous and had hot flashes. It was really happening for her. She grew more and more excited about every symptom when one hot day while helping to feed the animals she bled. She couldn't believe it; all that pain, the secrets, and hard work. She needed that baby. "Mom, Dad, I'm having a miscarriage. I'm having a miscarriage," she screeched. They were in almost as much shock as their daughter was and quickly brought her to the hospital.

"How could she be pregnant? Where did we go wrong with her? How could we have let this happen?" her mom questioned. She went for an ultrasound and immediately to surgery. Her parents ultimately got their wish; their daughter lived but could never bear children.

SHAMMING DIDN'T NEVER HURT NOBODY

A girl was brought to the hospital via ambulance in a coma. She had been admitted previously because she became bulimic and anorexic. She lost a massive amount of weight but still saw no change in the mirror. This is a real thing. With a condition like this, you will still look the same in your mind, no matter how much weight you lose. She was doing this because a group of girls were making fun of her, because of her above average size. Now, my mom has always told me that it's ok to make fun of someone if it is something that they can go home and change the next day; as in bad makeup, smelly armpits, sweat-stains or cutting out your shirt sleeves as if the sleeves ran away from you, for instance. Even then, it's usually not ok unless you are friends and have a joking kind of relationship. Anything other than that is unacceptable. Even though the girl lost weight, the taunting never stopped. The girl was gorgeous and couldn't see past a group of mean girls. Her mom was diabetic and had her own medical issues to deal with. She did not understand this was going on, let alone controlling her life. The mother depended on her daughter for everything. That day she found her daughter lying on the floor with an empty insulin bottle. She was still alive. She was rushed to the hospital. That insulin wasn't your everyday, run of the mill insulin. That would have killed her on the spot. She took the longest acting one on the market. It didn't kill her immediately but the doctors could do nothing, death was inevitable. She had a long, painful passing. Even though her death was mourned, it was still welcomed so her body and mind would suffer no more. As for the mean girls; they were first charged in the beginning weeks as information came forth, but the charges increased shortly following her untimely demise. As for her mother; she had to sell everything they owned to take care of a fraction of the medical bills and her house was foreclosed on. She now resides on the streets. All parties involved lost something that day.

HAPPY FATHER'S DAY

A young woman came in alive in body but absent from her mind from a single car collision. She was brain-dead. There was talk of possible suicide due to a situation with her boyfriend and a text that was sent. Her father was a single parent and had devoted his entire life to his daughter and now he was alone and faced with some tough decisions. He graciously gave the ultimate gift by sacrificing the thing he loved most in this world. His cherished daughter was a kind and giving soul. She always told her dad she wanted to donate her organs if anything happened to her. He never in his wildest dreams thought he would live to see this day. It turns out that the earlier situation dealt with a jealous girl that couldn't let go. The bitter girl slipped into her hospital room posing as a close family member just as her dad left for only a moment. That moment was long enough to pull down her hospital sheets and take multiple pictures of her naked, vulnerable, lifeless body. She posted them on every major social media page she could to shame her. Mind you, she was literally just there to die as she could not be saved. The only reason she was still alive was for her father as it was Father's Day. This girl saved eight lives the next day. Her dad was so proud. He never let a tear drop through all of the pain and horror of the piled circumstances, until he went through her belongings. In her backpack laid a card meant for him only a day ago. In it she spoke of having such an amazing father and that she didn't want him to think any less of her. She continued saying she just discovered she was pregnant and couldn't wait for him to meet his grandchild. She said that she would love him no matter what, even past her dying day.

PART I OF II: BALLS FOR DAYS

A man had endured way too many bath salts amongst other things and came into the hospital to detox at the request of the police. He was physically aggressive and verbally abusive. I had him strapped up in restraints with a mask over his face to prevent him from spitting. He wanted to get out so badly he couldn't stand it and all he had was time on his hands. He continuously worked and worked and worked some more at getting out of the restraints. He finally got them loose enough they gave way. From there he unstrapped his ankles. He went for it. He ran out the door as fast as he could. An alarm sounded off coming from the bed. He had to think fast. He tried to get out the front double doors of the unit, but they were locked. He had to go another way. By this time, he created quite the stir amongst the overloaded, burnt out nurses. The hospital entourage was after him, but it didn't take much to get out from our clutches. I mean, what were we going to do anyway? Were we supposed to tackle him to the ground? We could not lay a hand on him. Plus he was utterly buck-booty naked. Security had been called but hadn't arrived. He was quick and in fight or flight mode. He wasn't thinking, just reacting; all he knew was that he needed to get out of there and fast. He saw a safety exit arrow for emergencies and followed the signs to a stairwell. Another alarm sounded once the door opened. He ran down the stairs as if his life depended on it. He made it to the bottom and out the emergency fire exit. He wasn't out of the woods yet, so he had to figure out a way to go as far and fast as he could. There was a parking lot straight across the street. At least there he would be safe and out of reach from the out of shape security guards. If anyone stood in his way, he would have to fight. And that he did. He fought three people on the way, attempting to pull another person out of their car. As you can imagine a grown man naked throwing fists and kicking is not a pretty site. It draws attention. As he removed the person from their vehicle, a math teacher came to the rescue and subdued him. He was charged and convicted for many years and I lost my license. That goes to show you that if someone has nothing to lose, that person can lose everything for you.

PART II OF II: BALLS FOR DAYS

A young man came in with a flesh-eating disease that traveled up his leg. I will never understand why people never come in to be seen until something like this reaches their private parts. Anyways, I had this patient three days in a row and I was busy that day. I was trying to rush through my assessment as he was healthy, but spent time where it counted which was on his wound. A bed alarm went off. I normally would go, but this day was unusually busy and if I was busy doing someone else's job, then mine would never get done. I finished my physical assessment and charted while I was in the room multitasking, giving meds and asking questions. Suddenly there was a strange flash of something that went by the open door. "That was strange," the patient said. Next thing we saw was the slowest moving herd of nurses you've ever seen saying, "No... stop... no... don't do it." They were seriously in slow motion. A new alarm sounded off coming from the stairwell. I couldn't be distracted and there looked to be plenty of help going towards the two continuous alarms going off. What could go wrong? In finishing up, the patient asked me if he could wash up. He had a wound VAC (a medical suction device that helps wounds to heal faster and prevent infection) that needed to be changed out by the wound care nurses later that day. I told him I would page them and find out if he could take a shower. It was yet another thing to add to my task list instead of taking things off that needed to be done before my shift was over. A few hours later, I was permitted to allow him to shower, but I had to unhook the wound VAC and hook it back in immediately after he finished showering. I noticed a big rush of powerful people come in. I went ahead and unhooked him as instructed for his shower, but he kept getting phone call after phone call. His friends heard on the news there was some naked man that escaped the hospital and was beating people up and immediately thought it was him. He finally went to the bathroom and got cleaned up while I tended to my other patients. He called me back in like he was supposed to so I could hook him back up. Being the prudent nurse I am, I removed the sterile caps I put on, connected the tubing back and turned the machine on. These machines start off at a low suction rate and cautiously go up in suction. I could hear the machine working but he wasn't getting any suction to his wound area. The machine worked harder, and the suction increased drastically on the machine trying to fix the problem and accommodate a possible air leak. The suction numbers kept going higher and higher even past the point where it would normally reside, but the patient still didn't have the slightest bit of a tug. He then brings to my attention that the clip on the tubing was still clamped down. Without thinking I quickly grabbed it out of his hand and unclamped it. I heard this major force of suction pressure followed by a bloodcurdling scream. Oh no, I'm generally so thorough. How could this have happened? It's like I've got fifteen hours' worth of work to do and only twelve hours to do it. Suddenly he yells at the top of his lungs, "My balls… you're sucking my balls off… you're sucking my balls off!" I had to get out of there and think so I bolted out quickly shutting the door behind me. He was still hollering about how I was still sucking his balls off. All the people were there that arrive when something big happens. Not that I don't enjoy brushing elbows with the bigwigs as much as the next guy but today was not the day. Someone was about to be fired and I was about to be on the firing range if he kept yelling. I grabbed several IV pain medication doses and came straight back. I immediately gave him the medicine and tried to calm him down and apologize. He shortly felt better and accepted my sincerest apologies. Once he cooled down, I went off to check on my other patients and get some charting done. As the bigwigs dispersed I got a minute to think about the situation and got upset. I stewed in it for a few minutes and couldn't take it anymore. I marched to his room, opened the door and exclaimed, "Great… now because of you, I have to go home, look my husband in the eye and tell him, 'Honey,

I'm sorry but I cheated on you... I sucked another man's balls off today!"

CALL FOR YOUR STORY

Do you have any interesting stories? Do you have something that you must get off your chest? Help me write my next book by emailing me at ArayahsunshineRN@gmail.com. Tell me what area of expertise you are in and what your thoughts are that you'd like to share. I want to see the world through your eyes. Please do not worry if I don't use your experience for the next volume, I may use it for a later edition and I will let you know. Some parts of the story may have to be changed for discretion. Keep it somewhat short and intriguing. If you will notice, there is more bad than good out there in this realm. I'd like something for each section, but I would really like to hear the good things. These are the reasons we do this; these are the reasons we are in this profession in the trenches with our patients. It gives us purpose and a reason to get up in the morning and hold our heads high. It would be nice if people from all over the world came together to share and to vent. See your story, ideas or situation in my next book. I'm open to all suggestions. If you'd like me to add you to my email list when you have a question please let me know. And yes, this is my real email so feel free to contact me and I will get back to you.

www.ingramcontent.com/pod-product-compliance
Lightning Source LLC
Chambersburg PA
CBHW031924240526
45464CB00022B/688